Advances in Modern
Environmental Toxicology

VOLUME III

ASSESSMENT OF REPRODUCTIVE AND TERATOGENIC HAZARDS

EDITED BY

MILDRED S. CHRISTIAN, Ph.D.
Argus Research Laboratories, Inc.

WAYNE M. GALBRAITH, Ph.D.
U.S. Environmental Protection Agency
Washington, D.C.

PETER VOYTEK, Ph.D.
U.S. Environmental Protection Agency

MYRON A. MEHLMAN, Ph.D.
Mobil Oil Corporation
Princeton, N.J.

Published by
Princeton Scientific Publishers Inc.
Princeton

Printed and bound in the United States of America.

PRINCETON SCIENTIFIC PUBLISHERS, INC.
P.O. Box 3159, Princeton, NJ 08540

LIBRARY OF CONGRESS 82-062165
ISBN 0-911131-03-5

Advances in Modern Environmental Toxicology Series: ISSN 0276-5063
ISBN 0-911131-00-0

Cover Art: Adapted from E.M. Johnson, p. 85.

EDITORIAL BOARD

M.R. Parkhie, D.V.M., Ph.D.
U.S. Food and Drug Administration

Michael A. Pereira, Ph.D.
U.S. Environmental Protection Agency

William R. Pool, Ph.D.
G.D. Searle & Co.

Leonard D. Saslaw, Ph.D.
United States Food and Drug Administration

B.V. Rama Sastry, D. Sc., Ph.D.
Vanderbilt University

Russell P. Sherwin, M.D.
University of Southern California
    Medical Center

Andrew Sivak, Ph.D.
Arthur D. Little, Inc.

Edward A. Smuckler, Ph.D., M.D.
University of California, San Francisco,
    School of Medicine

B.L. VanDuuren, Sc.D.
New York University Medical Center

Jerry R. Williams, D. Sc.
George Washington University
    Medical Center

TABLE OF CONTENTS

INTRODUCTION TO SECTIONS I AND II vii

SECTION I

CHAPTER 1 Statement of Problem
M.S. Christian.. 1

CHAPTER 2 The 1980's: An Era of Reproductive Confrontation
J.E. Goeke.. 5

CHAPTER 3 Pharmaceuticals, Drugs and Birth Defects
R.M. Hoar 13

CHAPTER 4 Foods, Food Additives and Natural Products
G. Nolen 19

CHAPTER 5 Petroleum and Petroleum Products: A Brief Review
of Studies To Evaluate Reproductive Effects
C. A. Schreiner.. 29

CHAPTER 6 Reproductive Toxicology: Radiation Effects
R.P. Jensh 47

CHAPTER 7 The Teratologist as a Consultant
E.M. Johnson 61

CHAPTER 8 Assessment of Reproductivity Toxicity: State of the Art
M.S. Christian.. 65

CHAPTER 9 Practical Application of Systems for Rapid
Detection of Potential Teratogenic Hazards
E.M. Johnson 77

SECTION II

Assessment of Risk to Human Reproduction and to
Development of the Human Conceptus from Exposure
to Environmental Substances 93iii

Table of Contents.............................. v

About the Series Editor......................... 160

INTRODUCTION

Man's survival depends on his ability to carry out normal reproduction from generation to generation. In this highly complex century, he is continually striving to improve the quality of his life through the development of new drugs and chemicals. The potential adverse effects of introducing these substances into man's environment, and the levels of exposure sufficient to produce these effects, are the concerns of reproductive toxicology.

This volume, *Assessment of Reproductive and Teratogenic Hazards,* is divided into two sections. The first, consists of nine chapters and includes a statement of the problem, an overview of historical perspectives, and a discussion of major incidents that have raised concern about reproductive hazards.

Additional chapters deal with reproductive hazards from environmental substances, pharmaceuticals, radiation, and food additives and with practical applications of systems for rapid detection of potential teratogenic hazards.

The second section was developed by a number of reproductive toxicologists and teratologists and has been critically reviewed and revised to cover the latest knowledge in these fields. It comprises five chapters and is entitled "Assessment of Risks to Human Reproduction and to Development of the Human Conceptus from Exposure to Environmental Substances."

Chapter Two of this section describes in detail a variety of toxicity and screening tests available to assess risk to female reproduction. Reproductive hazards to males are examined in Chapter Three. Chapter Four explores the current state of knowledge on estimation of risk to human conceptus from environmental substances. The last chapter covers epidemiology, pharmacokinetics, sexual behavior and priority areas for future research.

It is important to emphasize that extreme caution should be applied in extrapolating to human beings results obtained from animal experiments. The information presented in this book, within the limitations imposed by toxicology's heavy reliance on animal testing, should be of considerable value to toxicologists, teratologists, and biological scientists in government and industry who are concerned with the evaluation and assessment of reproductive hazards to men and women.

Myron A. Mehlman

SECTION I

CHAPTER 1

STATEMENT OF PROBLEM

Mildred S. Christian, Ph.D.
Argus Research Laboratories, Inc.
2025 Ridge Road
Perkasie, Pennsylvania 18944

PURPOSE

The purpose of this paper is to:

1. present the various types of reproductive hazards;
2. present the current scientific, economic and legal problems and influences on the field; and
3. present and describe the relevancy of both "state of the art" and developing methodology in reproductive toxicology.

Reproductive toxicology can be defined as the hazard to three populations at risk, the male, the female and the conceptus, each of which has distinct differences in toxic response and susceptibility.

Although most of the information presented is for use in consideration of the human risk potential, it must be remembered that other species also have potential reproductive risks. Since all species are relevant to our ecosystem, the relative risks to the entire ecosystem must be considered.

The three vertebrate populations at risk, regardless of species, are the male, the female, both gravid and non-gravid, and the conceptus.

TYPES OF REPRODUCTIVE HAZARD

Reproductive hazard to the male is usually perceived as decreased ability to perform the sexual act, morphologic change of sex organs, and/or decreased fertility as the result of reduced gamete production, reduced gamete viability and/or production of abnormal gametes. Fertility hazards in the female are similar to those in the male, but in addition include pregnancy, during which the female has different susceptibilities. The conceptus is at risk from long before birth, and the risk persists long after birth.

The following description of various parameters that potentially may be altered by toxic agents will demonstrate the multiplicity and complexity of the potential reproductive hazards.

A toxic response of gametogenesis can result in production of defective cells, cells which have heritable changes (mutagenicity) or changes in normal development. The duration of gametogenesis is significantly different in males and females. In the male, spermatogenesis requires approximately 60 days for the full cycle. In the female, only one complement of ova are produced during the entire lifespan. These ova develop to metaphase during the fetal stage in the female and remain at this stage of development until ovulated when the female is sexually mature.

Germ cell transport is susceptible to toxic effects. Transport may be affected by alteration of smooth muscle motility. The normal secretions of either the male or female genital tracts can be changed. Toxic agents may even enter these secretions and possibly affect the conceptus by direct exposure via these secretions.

The pregnant woman is at risk and more vulnerable to toxic agents during gestation because of physical, physiological and biochemical alterations from her non-pregnant state. Not only is the gravid female less able to perform such simple physical activities as easily rising from a chair, but more subtle changes exist which increase her susceptibility to toxic agents. Events such as the development of abnormal metabolic pathways, alteration of protein, carbohydrate and lipid metabolism, appetite suppression and augmentation, and the various changes in endocrine balance associated with the maintenance of the pregnancy may alter her susceptibility to toxic agents. Changes in maternal susceptibility are interrelated to the potential hazard for the conceptus.

Teratology, the field most frequently associated with reproductive toxicity, is actually concerned only with alteration of the conceptus. With the development of new endpoints for use in evaluations of assessment of teratogenic risk, just as it is now difficult to define the exact time at which death occurs, it is similarly difficult to define the time period during which teratogenic hazard exists. This inability to define exact endpoints for anatomical, physiological and "behavioral" teratogenic effects reflects the fact that the organ systems of the conceptus continue to develop and grow not only after primary morphological development has occurred but also after birth.

Toxins can alter maternal lactation and the response of the neonate. Not only may suckling be inhibited in the neonate, but the amount of available milk may be augmented or inhibited. The milk may be made unpalatable, or it may be toxic, as the result of presence of either the primary agent or its metabolites.

TIMING

When does hazard exist?

In the conceptus and neonate, both male and female reproductive development may be delayed and capacity altered. Behavioral and overt pathology have been reported. Sexually mature humans are at risk their entire reproductive lives.

METHOD OF EXPOSURE

How does exposure occur?

For adult humans, exposure can be classified as voluntary and involuntary. For the conceptus, all exposure is voluntary.

Voluntary exposure includes all hazards to which a person knowingly exposes him or herself, such as pharmaceuticals, radiation procedures and toxins in the home and workplace.

Involuntary exposure, a good portion of which is thought of as voluntary, includes all environmental pollutants, accidental exposure to toxins in the home or workplace, exposure to unrecognized toxins, and even such uncontrollable agents as weather and war.

The legal ramifications of voluntary versus involuntary exposure must be considered. For example, voluntary sterilization of a man or a woman is far different from involuntary sterilization following exposure to a toxin in the workplace or environment. Sterilization of a conceptus *in utero,* as has been reported in diethylstilbesterol-exposed humans, presents complex social and legal problems.

SCIENTIFIC, ECONOMIC AND LEGAL INFLUENCES ON REPRODUCTIVE TOXICOLOGY

Why are reproductive hazards now of interest?

The current interest reflects both the level of hazard and public awareness of the hazard. With improved lifestyles, new procedures and products have become potential hazards, new social concerns are present and the art of government regulation has been finetuned.

The public has become aware of an association of congenital malformations with both pharmaceutical and environmental agents. It remembers approximately 7,000 children with phocomelia resulting from maternal consumption of thalidomide. It remembers that *in utero* exposure to DES resulted in young adult women with vaginal adenocarcinomas and young men with testicular inclusion cysts and decreased fertility. It remembers misuse of the therapeutic agents aminopterin, as an abortificent, and progestional agents, as antiabortives, both resulting in malformed offspring. It questions the use of dilatin, an agent currently considered to be a weak teratogen and notes withdrawal syndromes in neonates exposed to morphine. It worries about the contamination of the environment with pollutants both from processing of chemical agents and from their use, and the possible risk associated with exposure to these agents. The public is pressing for legal protection from risk.

Although the public is aware, it not truly concerned that its own level of economic requirements for maintenance of its lifestyle, and its own drug-orientation (alcohol, smoking, drug addition), are intrinsic causes of the risks from which it wishes to be protected.

The ultimate purpose of this paper is to emphasize the importance of educating scientists, legislators, manufacturers and the general public about all of the known reproductive hazards which exist and the relative importance of these hazards. Included in this education is recognization that the economic need for new synthetic products and byproducts, the changes in and expectations of lifestyle and the relative risk resulting from maintaining that current level of human existence are interdependent. The entire population must be more aware of the ramifications of the requirements that may be placed on industry, the self-gratification which must be denied in order to live with these requirements, and the relative risk associated with continuence or improvement of its lifestyle.

CHAPTER 2

THE 1980's: AN ERA
OF REPRODUCTIVE CONFRONTATION

Jane E. Goeke, M.A.
Coordinator of Quality Assurance,
Argus Research Laboratories, Inc.
Instructor of History,
Community College of Philadelphia

INTRODUCTION

It is fitting that Americans have developed a pervasive sense of concern about the problems of reproductive toxicology in this, the last quarter of the 20th century. It is, after all, almost 25 years since the Minamata disaster, 20 years since the thalidomide tragedy and 10 years since the horrifying discovery of the delayed carcinogenic effects of DES (Diethylstilbestrol). The voices of anxiety, reform and even panic now echo from the corridors of academic, labor, industry, women's rights establishments, the law courts and, lately, even from the cavernous halls of the federal government.

The general consensus of opinion in the scientific community, as reflected by a recent spate of publications and meetings on the subject of reproductive toxicity, is that no one really knows enough about the subject to make definitive judgements or recommendations. As one researcher noted in 1976, "We are living in a sea of chemicals that have not been tested for their ability to cause cancer and birth defects," and, one might add, genetic mutations. A labor leader recently dubbed the 1980's the "decade of genetic confrontation" (2), an appellation with which several major chemical and pharmaceutical industries would doubtless agree, since they are currently facing lawsuits for reproductive and teratogenic damage allegedly incurred by their employees while on the job. The primary response of women's rights organizations to this reproductive crisis has focused on the apparent collision of two social goals; the right of all American women to equal employment opportunity, and the right of all American children to a safe, unpolluted fetal environment. A popular womens' magazine recently asked, "Are dangerous substances in the workplace in fact more hazardous to pregnant women then to other workers, specifically men" (3)? **Are all** women of childbearing age to be penalized because they "have this peculiarity: They are the childbearers of the race" (3)? The legal profession is also confused as to how it is to insure, conterminably, the rights of the human female and the human conceptus. In addition, the law is mired in conceptions of legal liability which developed in a simpler age of limited but direct and immediate environmental poisoning. A coherent body of case law which would delineate blame and compensation in cases involving the indirect and sometimes delayed effects of environmental teratogens, mutagens and transplacental carcinogens has yet to take shape.

Finally, inevitably, the federal government has entered the fray by proposing guidelines - soon to become regulations - on employment discrimination and reproductive hazards, and on the scope and precise nature of future research requirements (4). There can be no doubt that the era of reproductive confrontation has truly arrived. Members of the scientific community, despite a humble willingness to admit their limitations in the face of human complexity and universal infinity, are notably ahistorical. They practice their art - and art it is despite their pretensions of objectivity - as if it had no relationship to, and did not grow out of temporal social, economic and political conditions. While scientists are certainly willing to admit that their accomplishments are built upon the research and models of their predecessors, they seem blithely unaware of the fact that whole areas of research, in fact whole bodies of scientific knowledge come into being not because they are true or logical or useful, but because they are socially acceptable, politically correct and economically profitable. And for the very same reasons, many kinds of knowledge are ignored; ignored, that is, until the time is ripe for them.

An example of this historical truism with which you might be familiar involves the timing of the discovery of America. Why did Europe react with such interest, such energy, such an explosion of exploration, conquest and settlement at Columbus' discovery of America in 1492, when in fact the Vikings had already discovered and colonized parts of North America in the 12th century? Briefly and simplistically put, because Europe in 1492 was ready for such a discovery. In 1100, Europe did not seek a profitable route to trade with the Indies; in 1500, it did. In 1100, Europe did not believe it had excess population; in 1500, it did. In 1100, Europe did not possess the technology to easily sail the Atlantic; in 1500, it did. In 1100, Europe was mired in the dark ages and had a rather limited sense of progress; in 1500, having experienced the Renaissance and the Reformation, Europe had an unlimited vision of human possibilities.

The historical model I have suggested here is equally valid in the development of knowledge about and concern with the problems of reproductive toxicology. It is instructive that the branches of medicine devoted to the care of the human young, obstetrics and pediatrics, did not develop until after Western Civilization developed a conception of childhood as a separate and distinct state of human development, until after the sentimentalization of childhood led to an appreciation of children as separate individuals rather than a mass of "innocent vipers" (5). In a sense, teratology with its emphasis on the new preventative medical concept of prenatal mothering (6), is the culmination of that centuries long movement. The new awareness of children and childhood as something special has now been extended backwards through the fetal sojourn and even to the embryonic experience of the parent organism. It is equally instructive that a widespread concern with toxicology, in any form, is not prevalent in the Western world until the industrial revolution, until the factory, in creating the modern world also created the polluted world. The age of plenty has come to mean not only the prevalence of material goods and services, but also the prevalence of new illnesses and new possibilities for human destruction.

THE RELATIONSHIP OF REPRODUCTIVE TOXICOLOGY TO THE INDUSTRIALIZATION AND THE FEMINIZATION OF WORK

The genesis of reproductive toxicology, as a social concern and as a science, can be attributed to three developments in the history of the United States. The first and most significant of these is 19th century industrialization and its corollary, the movement of large numbers of women into the workforce. The second is the evolution of experimental mammalian teratology as a science and the third concerns the progression of the concept of legal liability from a mere contractual obligation to an ethical and moral requirement. The culmination and confluence of these three broad trends has occurred in this last quarter of the twentieth century.

Even the most ancient references to reproductive hazards are sex and process specific in that they are usually focused on the female and on the possibilities of teratogenesis. In Judges 13:7 of the Bible, the woman is admonished, "Behold thou shalt conceive and bear a son: and drink no wine or strong drink" (7). In classical Greece, Aristotle noted, "Foolish, drunken and hairbrained women most often bring forth children like unto themselves, morose and languid" (7). But it is not until the advent of the modern work environment, the physical and psychological separation of work place and home place, the development of the factory and mass production as social and economic realities, that scientific concern with reproductive hazards threatening the female population become paramount and systematic.

The first evidence of this development occurs in Victorian America during the 1870's and the 1880's, a time of violent and explosive industrialization and urbanization. Amusingly enough, Victorian physicians were little concerned about the filth, pollution and overwork which constituted the working environment of most women of the period, but rather with the fact that old social values, especially those which decreed that the woman's place was in the home, were being challenged (8). These concerned

M.D.'s were not long in discovering the terrible price women would have to pay for their new mobility and freedom. The "mannish maidens" (8) of the Victorian workplace were doomed to an existence permeated with anxiety, hysteria, and depression, not to mention sexual dysfunction (8) "mannish maidens" lost their sex drive, produced few and inferior children and often became sterile. An even more potent reproductive hazard than work was to be found in the education of women. One supposedly conclusive study on this subject demonstrated that of 705 Victorian women who had gone to college, only 196 married, only 66 had children, and a high % of this latter group suffered stillbirths (8). As one Alabama physician histrionically admonished.

> "Women beware. You are on the brink of destruction. You have hitherto engaged in crushing your waists; now you are attempting to cultivate your mind: You have been merely dancing all night in the foul air of the ballroom; now you are beginning to spend your mornings in study. You have been incessantly stimulating your emotions with concerts and operas, with French plays, and French novels; now you are exerting your understanding to learn Greek, and solve propositions in Euclid. Beware. Science pronounces that the woman who studies is lost." (8)

I have chosen this apparently silly episode in American medicine because it demonstrates two trends in the history of reproductive toxicology which are venerable and constant. First, the social concern with reproductive hazards appears only when women enter the workplace in relatively large numbers. Second, the medical and managerial response to this development has been rather consistently to bar the women from the workplace, based always, of course, on ostensibly rational, empirical perfectly objective grounds.

Despite the prejudices and pronouncements of Victorian medico's, the drift of American women into the workplace has been irreversible, if at times a bit dilatory. Three times during the 20th century, that movement has become a flood, and each time it has evoked new and more powerful responses to the dangers of reproductive hazards, first in the workplace, then in the environment as a whole.

The first of these hightides of female employment crests during World War I. In order for the United States to win the first of her foreign military victories through superior technology and productivity factories had to expand and proliferate. Yet at the same time the American workforce was contracted and decimated by the call to arms. The solution to this quandry was simple and predictable; let women man the workfront while men fought the war.

One must also recall that some 15 years prior to this "war to end all wars" (9), 1900 to be precise, Americans entered a period of pervasive reform known as Progressivism. Defined most simplistically, Progressivism meant an optimistic belief in grass roots democracy and the ability of the people to run their affairs successfully. The unholy alliance between corrupt political power and big business was to be broken and the lives of all Americans, but especially the poor and underprivileged, were to be improved. This reform impulse is relevant to the present discussion in that it provided the impetus for a general movement to improve working conditions in the United States, most especially a clean up of the innumerable toxic workplaces. During this period a new type of doctor, first produced by Johns Hopkins School of Medicine, became the American ideal: the expertly trained physician who was also a highly motivated social reformer (10). From this group came the first of the really competent industrial physicians (10), and the first of the really gifted teachers for the new branch of industrial medicine and the new science of industrial toxicology. It seems fair to say then, that Progressivism awoke Americans to the toxicity of their work environment at the same time that the entry of large numbers of female workers into war industries exacerbated these new perceptions.

The first researcher of real renown in the field of reproductive toxicology in the United States was Dr. Alice Hamilton, who also happens to have been the first woman ever appointed to the Harvard medical faculty. A reform minded physician, she began her work as the first American specialist in industrial diseases. Her publications are endless, and include monographs on industrial toxicology in the production of paint, storage batteries, sanitary ware and munitions (11). As a result of her efforts, the first state commissions on occupational diseases were established, workman's compensation was extended to include industrial poisoning, and many work places were cleaned up, at least to the extent of providing washrooms, protective clothing, separate eating facilities and better ventilation (10).

Dr. Hamilton's claim to fame in the field of reproductive toxicology is simple; she was the first scientist to assert that certain chemicals might be more hazardous for the unborn child than they were for the adult worker. This realization grew out of her work on women in industry, and is reflected in her path breaking publication, *Women in the Lead Industries,* 1919 (12). Female workers who suffer from lead poisoning, she noted, are "more likely to be sterile or to have miscarriages and stillbirths than are women not exposed to lead. If they bear living children these are more likely to die during the first year of life than are the children of women who have never been exposed to lead. This means that lead is a race poison, and that lead poisoning in women affects not only one generation, but two generations" (12). Later on, as she did in her work on carbon monoxide poisoning, Dr. Hamilton also came to the conclusion that substances mildly or nontoxic to the mother, could be deadly for the developing conceptus (13).

Dr. Hamilton's work was sex specific in that she only saw danger to the fetus through maternal teratogenesis, and place specific in that she identified only the workplace as hazardous to fetal health. Her solution to the problem, to bar women from certain industries and/or jobs, was followed only in the most inconsistent way between the wars (14). Although only two states barred women from working in lead related industries (15), most states barred them from working with moving machinery (where they might have their hands crushed, but then so could a man) or from working in dusty places (where their lungs might be harmed, but then so could a man's) (15). In short, the exclusion of women from the workplace between the World Wars was based more on sexual bias than sexual science, and was often used as an excuse not to clean up the workplace.

World War II again brought countless American women into industry and business, but the response to this phenomenon in the field of reproductive toxicology was negligible. As usual, when women became necessary to American productivity, the barriers to their employment came down, but the end of the war found most American females of reproductive age where they were supposed to be; at the center of home and hearth. One female physician, Dr. Anna Baetjer, did write a rather unique book called *Women in Industry* in which she attempted to critically examine if not demolish some of the old myths about working women, but her chapters on "Gynecological and Obstetrical Problems Associated with the Employment of Women" (16), and "Mortality and Fertility of Women in Relation to Occupation" (16), are more a plea for understanding than an authoritative statement. These sections were included, she notes, "not so much in the hope of presenting information...but rather to point out the need for investigation in this field and to serve as a word of caution in interpreting the data available at present" (16).

The contemporary surfeit of women in the American workplace cannot, for once, be attributed to war time conditions. Equal opportunity legislation, the civil rights movement, the feminist drive, inflation, the self awareness mystique have all played a part in creating this condition. What is unique about this flood of working women is that it promises not to peak in the immediate future; it seems to be a permanent rather than a transient development. But it has occurred at a time when America's image of itself is shifting from a land of limitless plenty to a domain of riches which are diminishing and must be carefully used and hoarded, from a country which could endlessly absorb waste and overuse to an ecologically finite commonwealth. And, it has occurred at a time when we have not only the nuclear potential to destroy the world many times over, but also the more time consuming ability to poison ourselves and our offspring for generations to come with the 73,000 untested chemicals and drugs we already have, not to mention the 2,000 new ones we invent annually (17). It is hardly surprising, therefore, that we have entered the era of publications such as "Guidelines on Pregnancy and Work" (18), "Nuclear Macho" (19), and "What We Must Know About Hazards in the Workplace" (3). We have also entered an age of Symposia with themes like "Occupational Health and Safety" (20), "Drugs and Chemical Risks to the Fetus and Newborn" (6), and our own "Reproductive Toxicology Workshop". As a social concern, reproductive toxicology has come of age. In recognition of that fact, it has received the ultimate accolade of our times; it has been popularized. Lonely American heroes like the "Rebel Without A Cause", the "Godfather", and the "Electric Horseman", must now share the stage with the "Elephant Man".

REFERENCES

1. McCann, J. and Ames, B.N.: Annual NY Acad. Sci., 1967.
2. Rawls, R.L.: CEN, February 11, 1980, 28.
3. Edmiston, S. and Szekely, J.: Redbook, March 1980, 33, 171.
4. "Interpretive Guidelines on Employment Discrimination and Reproductive Hazards", Federal Register, Friday, February 1, 1980, Part VI, Equal Employment Opportunity Commission; Department of Labor, 41 CFR Part 60-20.
5. Stannard, D.E.: Centuries of Childhood, New York, Vintage Books, 1962.
6. Smith, D.W., M.D.: Drugs and Chemical Risks to the Fetus and Newborn, eds., Schwarz and Haffe, 1980, 73.
7. Warner, R.H. and Rosett, H.L.: J. Stud. Alc 36, 1975, 1395.
8. Haller, J.S. and Haller, R.M.: The Physician and Sexuality in Victorian America, 1974, 29, 28, 29, 38-39, 39.
9. Zinn, H.: A People's History of the United States, 1980, 355.
10. Taylor, L.C., Jr.: The Medical Profession and Social Reform, 1885-1945, 1974, 6.
11. Hamilton, A.: "Hygiene of the Painters Trade", "Lead Poisoning in the Manufacture of Storage Batteries", "Lead Poisoning in the Potteries, Tile Works and Porcelain Enameled Sanitary Ware Factories", and "Industrial Poisons Used in the Manufacture of Explosives", in various Bulletins of the United States Bureau of Labor Statistics, 1913, 1914, 1914, 1917.
12. Hamilton, A.: "Women in the Lead Industries", Bulletin of the United States Bureau of Labor Statistics, 11-12, 1919.
13. Hamilton, A.: "Carbon Monoxide Poisoning", Bulletin of the United States Bureau of Labor Statistics, 15-16, 1922.
14. Mettert, M.T.: "State Reporting of Occupational Disease", United States Department of Labor, Bulletin of the Women's Bureau, No. 114, Washington Government Printing Office, 12-15, 1934.
15. No author listed: "The Employment of Women in Hazardous Industries in the United States", United States Department of Labor, Bulletin #6, 7, 7-8, 1921.
16. Baetjer, A.: Women in Industry, 159-193, 213-244, 211, 1946.
17. Sloane, Shapiro and Mitchell: Drugs and Chemical Risks to the Fetus and Newborn, eds. Schwarz and Yaffe, 2, 1980.
18. "Guidelines on Pregnancy and Work": DHEW (NIOSH) Publication No. 78-118, August 1979.
19. Cunningham, A.M.: Savvy, August, 1980.
20. "Occupational Health and Safety Symposia": DHEW(NIOSH) Publication No. 77-179, 1977.

CHAPTER 3

PHARMACEUTICALS, DRUGS AND BIRTH DEFECTS

Richard M. Hoar, Ph.D.
Assistant Director
Head, Teratology

Department of Toxicology and Pathology
Hoffmann-La Roche Inc.
Nutley, New Jersey 07110

Although drugs play a relatively small role in the production of known birth defects in man, two considerations make them an important factor in any analysis of human malformations. First, in spite of all the warnings and adverse publicity, women are still being given prescribed drugs and taking self-prescribed medicines while pregnant thus continuing to expose their developing offspring to potential teratogens. Second, malformations associated with pharmaceuticals produce spectacular publicity which draws attention away from the true nature and depth of the problem, lulling the public into accepting simple explanations for an extremely complex question. Should the general public understand that less than 3 malformed children out of an expected 60 per 1000 live births are induced by pharmaceuticals, they would feel betrayed and disappointed for then they would have to accept how little science knows about birth defects and how much of the responsibility for them still remains with the public.

I do not intend to detail each pharmaceutical which is known or suspected of producing malformations in man, but instead I would like to provide you with a kaleidoscopic impression of the present scene organized with an eye to establishing responsibility. For example, responsibility for the thalidomide disaster rests squarely upon the deficiencies of the science at that time, its inadequate testing programs and our failure to understand how easy it is to confront the developing mammalian embryo with noxious stimuli. Several thousand crippled children, perhaps as many as 7000 infants, with defects primarily of the extremities and face, serve to remind teratologists that in 1961, when thalidomide was indicted, they were not using a satisfactory laboratory model or screening technique to examine compounds for their potential teratogenicity. Those who still remained to be convinced about the failure of the placenta to serve as a protective barrier for the developing child had their convictions shattered by the rubella epidemic in the United States in 1964 which resulted in almost 20,000 defective children (Schardein, 1976). We now know that almost any compound can cross the placenta particularly if it is of low molecular weight (Yaffee, 1979). As a result of these bitter lessons, the science of teratology has advanced, our complacency has been reduced and the need for constant vigilance in the form of improved epidemiologic surveillance has been accepted.

Pharmaceuticals are developed as adjuncts to therapeutic medicine and as such are employed with a specific result in mind. However, the activity of such compounds has occasionally been mis-directed at the developing conceptus resulting in unanticipated embryotoxicity which may be apparent either at birth or years later. Thus it was that in the early 1950's the association of the widespread use of synthetic progestational agents in cases of threatened abortion, with the masculinization of the female external genitalia *in utero* came as an unpleasant surprise. It became apparent that the degree of masculinization depended upon both the androgenic properties of the synthetic progestins and the extent of the treatment period; the differentiation of the external genitalia being essentially completed by the end of the twelfth week of gestation so that continued treatment after this date had little effect (Schardein, 1976; Wilson, 1977). Even more surprising was the association of diethylstilbestrol (DES), a non-steroidal estrogen, with the appearance of adenocarcinoma of the vagina and uterine abnormalities in young women (Bibbo, et al, 1975; Hill and Stern, 1979). Given during the 1950's and 1960's as a treatment for threatened abortions during the first trimester, the compound was not associated with prenatal damage to the developing offspring until twenty years later! Although not the first example of a prenatal insult producing an effect not seen until some time after birth, it certainly alerted the public to such a possibility! Fortunately, very few of the female fetuses so exposed developed an adenocarcinoma; however, the picture has been complicated further by the realization that young males similarly exposed *in utero* have a 25% incidence of epididymal cysts, hypotrophic testes, capsular induration of the testes and associated fertility problems (Bibbo, et al, 1975; Henderson, et al, 1976; Gill, et al, 1977, Globus, 1980).

We are not always surprised by the teratogenic activity of a drug, for on occasion its intended use is known not to be compatible with normal embryonic development. Thus the use of cancer chemotherapeutic agents during pregnancy is associated with a high risk of teratogenesis in animals and embryotoxicity in man. Compounds such as busulfan, chlorambucil, and cyclophosphamide are but three of the many alkylating agents implicated as human teratogens and expected to be on the basis of their chemical action (Schardein, 1976; Wilson, 1977). That these chemicals are given at close to the maximum tolerated dosage merely increases the risk of teratogenesis and the need for an informed public to avoid misunderstanding of their teratogenic potential.

Antimetabolites are effective anticancer agents also and as such are embryotoxins. Among them the folic acid antagonist, aminopterin, is a potent teratogen producing skull, limb and CNS anomalies. This is but one of several such compounds, exhibiting embryolethality in animal studies, that have been misused as abortifacients in humans with horrifying results (Schardein, 1976). Unfortunately there are too many variables in a human pregnancy, such as the stage of embryogenesis, drug susceptibility, metabolism, etc., to guarantee the action of these compounds as abortifacients and their use as such should be discontinued.

As therapeutic agents have produced expected as well as unexpected teratology, our experience with them has shown itself in a developing awareness of the teratogenic potential of any compound and an ever-increasing list of suspected teratogens. However, any association between drug and malformation must be examined critically for the defects could have ocurred spontaneously, be the result of the mother's genetic constitution, or due to the disease for which the drug was given. Anticonvulsants in general and diphenylhydantoin in particular are examples of both this increased focus of attention and the interference of the disease entity itself with any subsequent analysis. To simplify this discussion let us refer to the report of Janz (1975) who stated that defects among live births appeared with a frequency of 6.0% in epileptic mothers treated with anticonvulsants, 4.2% in nontreated epileptics, and 2.5% in mothers who were not epileptics. He concluded that the increased risk must be due at least in part to the disease itself. I would agree with his conclusion and suggest that only if he had been able to establish a group of untreated epileptic mothers whose disease was comparable in severity to that of the treated mothers (an obvious impossibility) could he have improved the conditions of his analysis. This inability to match subjects perfectly for an analysis is but one of the confounding factors encountered in epidemiology preventing an unencumbered analysis and an unbiased decision which explains why we presently accept the viewpoint that anticonvulsants are "weak" teratogens whose risk of producing a malformation is too small to recommend discontinuing treatment during pregnancy (Schardein, 1976).

We have been considering the association of birth defects with prescribed drugs and therapeutics. However, it was noted that pregnant women self-prescribe pharmaceutical products. In fact, based on a sample of 50,282 pregnancies, the mean number of these preparations taken has increased from 2.6 per pregnancy in 1958 to 4.5 in 1965 (Heinonen, et al, 1977) and Schardein (1976) has compiled a series of references which suggest even higher levels of self-medication. As difficult to understand as this may be in light of the repeated warnings to avoid any pharmaceuticals while pregnant, it is even more shocking to see birth defects arising from the use of drugs of abuse such as heroin, methadone, or alcohol.

The child born to a methadone or heroin addict will show signs of acute narcotic withdrawal at birth. In addition there are reports that these children exhibit central nervous system hyperirritability lasting for as long as 4-6 months and attention impairment, sometimes accompanied by hyperactivity, for 2-3 years. (For a review of these findings see Hutchings, 1978). Once again we have an example of delayed postnatal effects resulting from a prenatal insult. However, this does not involve a structural abnormality but rather a CNS defect which can only be assessed by measurement of behavioral modifications! Surely no one would be surprised to learn that the development of techniques for examining CNS damage in animals has become a major objective in teratology!

The fetal alcohol syndrome (FAS) is a good example of the teratologists' failure to couple understanding with the admonition against the consumption of any "drugs" during pregnancy. This syndrome resulting from excessive maternal alcohol consumption during pregnancy includes craniofacial, limb and cardiovascular defects coupled with prenatal growth retardation, mental deficiency and postnatal failure to thrive (Jones and Smith, 1973, 1975; Jones, et al, 1973; Jones et al, 1974). The actual number of these children is difficult to ascertain, but in light of the prevalence of alcoholics in our population, the potential is frightening!

Teratologists must continue to struggle with the development of their science, attempting to eliminate the "surprises" among the pharmaceuticals, warning everyone of the obvious teratogens and increasing the public's understanding of its responsibilities both to its unborn children and to each other through intensified epidemiologic surveillance. We should be reminded that birth defects are not always structural malformations seen at birth, but may appear much later as abnormal physiologic mechanisms or aberrant behavior patterns, etc. Remember also that the labelling of a substance as a teratogen by mere apposition of the compound and the defect, utilizing a small sample size, flouts epidemiologic principles (Heinonen, et al, 1977). To establish at a 95% confidence level that a particular drug increases the naturally occurring frequency of a congenital malformation by 1% would require a population sample of at least 35,000 pregnant women! Finally, we must foster the realization that drug abuse, and the birth defects resulting from it, is everyone's problem because it ranges from excess prescriptions of medicines to self-medication and includes alcoholism and the use of illicit drugs. We should accept responsibility for our own habits before we accuse others of endangering our unborn children.

REFERENCES

1. Bibbo, M., Al-Naqueeb, M., Baccarini, I., Gill, W., Newton, M., Sleeper, K., Sonek, M., and Wied, G.L.: Follow-up study of male and female offspring of DES-treated mothers - a preliminary report. J. Reprod. Med. 15: 29-32, 1975.
2. Gill, W.B., Schumacher, G.F.B., and Bibbo, M.; Pathological semen and anatomical abnormalities of the genital tract in human male subjects exposed to diethylstilbestrol in utero. J. Urol. 117: 477-480, 1977.
3. Globus, M.S.: Teratology for the obstetrician: current status. Obstet. Gynec. 55: 269-277, 1980.
4. Henderson, B.E., Benton, B., Cosgrove, M., Baptista, J., Aldrich, J., Townsend, D., Hart, W., and Mock, T.M.: Urogenital tract abnormalities in sons of women treated with diethylstilbestrol. Pediatrics 58: 505-507, 1976.
5. Heinonen, O.P., Slone, D., and Shapiro, S.; birth defects and drugs in pregnancy. Littleton, Mass., Publishing Sciences Groups, Inc., 1977.
6. Hill, R.M., and Stern, L.: Drugs in pregnancy: Effects on the fetus and newborn. Drugs 17: 182-197, 1979.
7. Hutchings, D.: Behavioral teratology: Embryopathic and behavioral effects of drugs during pregnancy. *In* Gottlieb, G. (Editor); *Various Influences on Brain and Behavioral Development.* New York, Academic Press, Inc., 1978, pp. 7-34.
8. Janz, D.: The Teratogenic risk of antiepileptic drugs. Epilepsia 16: 159-169, 1975.
9. Jones, K.L., and Smith, D.W.: Recognition of the fetal alcohol syndrome in early infancy. Lancet 2:999-1001, 1973.
10. Jones, K.L., and Smith, D.W.: The fetal alcohol syndrome. Teratology 12:1-10, 1975.
11. Jones, K.L., Smith, D.W., and Ulleland, C.J.: Pattern of malformation in offspring of chronic alcoholic mothers. Lancet 1:1267-1271, 1973.
12. Jones, K.L., Smith, D.W., Steissguth, A.P., and Myrianthopoulos, N.C.: Outcome in offspring of chronic alcoholic women. Lancet 1: 1076-1078, 1974.
13. Schardein, J.L.: Drugs as teratogens. Cleveland, CRC Press, 1976.
14. Wilson, J.C.: Embryotoxicity of drugs in man. *In* Wilson, J.G. and Fraser, F.C. (Editors): *Handbook of Teratology: Volume I General Principles and Etiology.* New York, Plenum Press, 1977, pp. 309-356.
15. Yaffee, J.S.: Drugs during pregnancy. Guidelines to Professional Pharmacy 2:2, 1979.

CHAPTER 4

FOODS, FOOD ADDITIVES
AND NATURAL PRODUCTS

Dr. Granville Nolen, A.B.
The Procter and Gamble Co.
Miami Valley Laboratory
P.O. Box 39175
Cincinnati, Ohio 45247

Reproductive toxicity caused by the diet is rare in humans. However, three cases demonstrate that the diet can be a vehicle for producing reproductive toxicity in man. Endemic cretinism that occurred in central Europe up until some thirty years ago, and which still occurs in a few small areas around the world is the result of iodine deficiency--a frank nutritional deficiency disorder due to a lack of iodine in soils and food (1). Minimata disease, which occurred in Japan a little more than 20 years ago, resulted from an environmental contaminant, methyl mercury, being sequestered and concentrated in the food chain, in this case, fish (2). Another example, is the retarded growth and sexual maturation (especially hypogonadism in males) seen in certain areas of the Middle East, due to zinc and iron disorders, brought about by excessive dietary copper or phytate (3).

Animal studies have shown that a number of food components, mostly occurring naturally as contaminants, can produce reproductive toxicity primarily teratogenicity (4). These include alkaloids, polypeptides, nutritional antagonists, and a wide variety of bacterial and fungal toxins occurring as contaminants of agricultural products (Table 1). In addition, deficiencies or excesses of vitamins and minerals, particularly vitamin A, can interrupt reproduction or produce embryolethality and abnormal development (1). However, none of these toxicities have been observed in humans.

Only a very few food additives added intentionally during processing have ever been shown to cause reproductive toxicity in animals. EDTA, a chelating agent (5), and dioctyl sodium sulfosuccinate (6), an emulsifier, have been shown to be teratogenic in rats, but only at doses many hundreds of times greater than the human exposure levels. Although sodium cyclamate, saccharin and the food dye Red 2 (4) have been purported to

19

TABLE 1   Natural Substances Teratogenic In Animals

Material	Species
Locoweed	Sheep, Cattle
Lupins	Cattle
Wild Cherry	Swine
Chick Peas	Cattle, Sheep, Rat
Sweet Peas	Baboon
Tobacco Stalks	Swine
Bracken Fern	Mouse
Podophyllin	Mouse, Rat, Sheep
Aflatoxin	Mouse, Hamster
Ochratoxin	Mouse
Ergotamine	Mouse, Rat, Rabbit
Antibiotics from Molds	Various

1. From Ref. No. 4

cause either teratogenicity and/or embryolethality in animals, the data were not confirmed in later, better designed studies. See Reference 7 for an example. None of these materials have been associated with human reproductive toxicities.

The phthalate esters are examples of an unintentional food aditive that has been shown to be teratogenic in animals at high doses (8) but are of little concern to humans because the levels migrating to foods can be controlled to toxicologically insignificant amounts.

This history of cases shows that reproductive toxicity can be caused by foods, and warrants our continued vigilance in screening dietary components for such toxicities.

Although nutritional toxicology, including reproductive toxicology, involves the same principles and many of the techniques used in non-food toxicology, there are several special considerations in designing these studies owing to the overlap into the nutrition area. These will be the subject of this discussion.

It should go without saying, but you need to know the structure and something about the chemistry of the test material. Usually this is acquired during the course of its development as a potential food or food additive. Then come the simple acute tests, such as the oral LD50. However, some modification may be needed in testing food materials, because the LD 50 of a new major food component may be greater than the animal's intestinal capacity. For example, the LD50 in rodents of most vegetable oils is greater than 80 ml/kg (9). Therefore, a better acute test, depending on the nature of the material, might be a 3-10 day bioassay.

As soon as possible, the matabolism of the material, at least the absorption, distribution, and excretion patterns, needs to be determined. This is needed to show the systemic load at a number of dose levels, pin-point target organs, and determine similarities in handling between the animal and ultimately Man.

All of you have heard that the appropriate way to dose the material is the same as the route of human exposure. This is true for a safety study. However, this early in the safety network plan, we are attempting to determine the toxicity of the material. Along with the procedure of giving very high doses to intensify the effect, we may give the doses to animals in an unrealistic manner, such as IV or IP, to achieve the same end--that is, to determine the symptomatology of the materials toxicity. However, as we move forward in our toxicity--safety network, the methods of dosing, in general, should begin to be modeled after the route of human exposure.

With food materials, the normal route of administration is oral. But, should it be done by gavage or should it be a part of the diet? Gavage is usually easier, and at least for a short time, allows for a more closely controlled dose, but it causes stress on the animal, and more importantly delivers the material as a bolus, which may simply overwhelm the metabolic processes. In addition, intubation accidents are not infrequent and the resulting morbidity and mortality can seriously confound an experiment. Therefore, unless some circumstance dictates otherwise, the vehicle for a food safety study should be the diet. This vehicle delivers the test material in a more normal physiological way and places no undue stress on the animal. With reasonable care the amount delivered can be controlled and measured almost as precisely as with a gavaged dose.

Once it has been decided that diet will be the vehicle for the test material, the type of diet must be chosen; either a natural type diet, usually obtained commercially, or a semi-purified (also, semi-synthetic) diet. The cereal-based commercial types are fine for studies involving some additives and contaminants at levels which will not materially affect nutrient balances. They also are very stable with a long-shelf life and the nutrients in them are packaged in an organic matrix more like that consumed by the human. However, the cereal based-diets have varying levels of micro-nutrients, which may confound a study of a particular food or additive, such as an amino acid or trace mineral. Morever, the fat source and fatty acid composition may be uncertain, since animal feeds contain vegetable and animal fats from a variety of by-product sources. Therefore, a semi-purified diet, that can be purchased from supply houses or preferably made in the laboratory and whose composition can be very closely controlled, is recommended for most food or food additive studies.

A typical semi-purified diet, one recently recommended by a special committee of the American Institute of Nutrition (10), as a means of standardizing this type of diet is shown in Table 2. Note that they call the diet "purified" and recommend the usage of that term, although most nutritionists reserve that term for a diet containing mixtures of amino acids, rather than intact proteins. Casein, supplies the protein--it typically runs from 80-90% protein; the methionine is added to balance the amino acid

---

TABLE 2   Ain-76[TM]   Purified Diet For Rats And Mice

Ingredient	% By Weight
Casein	20.0
DL-Methionine	0.3
Cornstarch	15.0
Sucrose	50.0
Fiber	5.0
Corn Oil	5.0
AIN Mineral Mix	3.5
AIN Vitamin Mix	1.0
Choline Bitartrate	0.2
	100.0

1. From Ref. No. 10

---

profile, since casein is somewhat limiting in this essential amino acid. Cornstarch and sucrose furnish the carbohydrate, but various other proportions of complex and simple carbohydrates can be used. The fiber is added usually as cellulose, but others such as pectins or mucilages can be substituted if desired for experimental purposes.

Fat, except for essential fatty acids, is not required by the rat and the basal diet has a low level similar to commercial diets. The mineral and vitamin mixtures are formulated based on the National Research Counsel requirements for rodents (11).

A fairly typical semi-purified diet used in my laboratory is shown in Table 3. The list of major nutrients is the same as for the AIN diet, but the fat level has been increased to 20%, a sizeable increase. This is done because the human consumes a diet containing about 20% fat (40% of total calories). However, when the fat level is increased, which increases the caloric density of the diet, the protein level must be increased and you must be certain that the vitamins and minerals are adequate at the reduced feed intake. This is just one example of the consideration given the designing of the composition of the diet. Others are: Is the test material a new food or major dietary component? These may be either of some natural origin, or manmade. They may be minimally or highly processed. Or, is it some type of food additive that will occur only in trace amounts in the finished product, and in the total diet of the consumer?

First, we will consider some of the problem areas with new foods or major dietary components. One of the abiding rules in toxicology, is to feed or dose with exaggerated doses to establish effect-no effect levels. Since, for food materials, an acceptable human daily intake is generally set at 1/100th of the no-effect level in the animal study, we try to develop an anticipated human exposure and feed or dose the animals one dose level which is 100 times this amount. However, with a major nutrient this is clearly impossi-

TABLE 3   Typical Semi-Purified Diet

Ingredient	% By Weight
Casein	27.0
DL-Methionine	0.5
Cornstarch	20.0
Sucrose	24.5
Fiber	3.0
Mineral Mix	4.0
Vitamin Mix	1.0
Fat Or Oil	20.0
	100.0

ble. Nor, is it always needed, since the safety factor for many nutrients is much less. For example, the optimal amount of the sulfur amino acid, methionine, is about 0.5% of the diet, while simply doubling the level can produce toxicity (12). Depending upon the total dietary protein this leads to a safety factor of about 2 or 3. Similar low safety factors occur for the trace minerals, fat-soluble vitamins and for numerous naturally occurring toxicants in everyday foods.

Even a small exaggeration of one of the major food components can perturb the nutritional state of the animal leading to a disturbed physiological state, if not outright pathology. As I stated before, increasing the fat level can reduce feed intake, and an otherwise adequate diet can now become marginal, or even deficient for one or more nutrients including vitamins and minerals.

In Table 4, I have illustrated the diluting effects of increasing the fat level. Diet #1 designed with a 5% fat level, which will be consumed at the rate of 20 grams per day, will furnish the NRC nutrient requirements for the pregnant rat. However, by increasing only the fat level, leading to a reduced feed consumption, the diet is now limiting in many essential nutrients as shown here by these few examples. Dilution with other materials such as carbohydrate or fiber can lead to similar disturbances. The same sort of a problem can occur with a commercial type feed, where it is used as a basal diet and significant amounts of test material are added to it.

In addition to the induction of simple deficiencies one must be aware of altering several nutrient ratios, important for the animal's health. Some examples are shown in Table 5. The protein/calorie ratio, I've already touched upon; I'll come back to the calcium/phosphorus ratio later.

The ratio of saturated to polyunsaturated fatty acids has a wider latitude than I have indicated here, but it should receive some attention since, extremes in the ratio can affect absorption from the gut, and/or the stability of the diet. High levels of polyunsaturated fatty acids are extremely vulnerable to auto-oxidation, which can lead to the destruction of vitamins. Therefore, some special techniques, such as adding antioxidants and daily

TABLE 4

Nutrient	Diet#1	Diet#2
Fat Level, %	5	20
Lead/g	4	5
Feed Intake, g/day	20	16
Protein, g/day	3.8	3.0
Calcium, mg/day	120	96
Vitamin A, Iu/day	240	152
Thiamine, mg/day	.08	.06

TABLE 5   Important Nutrient Ratios

Nutrients	Recommended Ratio(s)
Prot/Cal	25-35 mg/Kcal
Ca/P	1.2-2.0:1
Fatty Acids, P/S	1:1
Amino Acids	Balanced Spectrum

feedings of fresh diet, are required. If an amino acid is the test material, then attention must be given to not only the absolute level, but also to the "balance" of the remaining amino acids. An animal can metabolize excessive amounts of a balanced protein, when similar excesses of only one or two amino acids can be quite toxic.

Food additives do not cause as many design problems as major nutrients, because their levels are generally quite low. Thus, they can be tested more like the usual chemical, including the use of commercial diets. However, the caveats mentioned earlier about nutritional perturbations apply here also, since many additives either are or contain essential trace nutrients. In addition, many others occur in the foods as salts, particularly Na and K (Table 6). Therefore, exaggerations based upon probable human exposures, or maximum tolerated doses, may induce the same sort of perturbations discussed earlier.

Table 7 illustrates a hypothetical, but very plausible case. Suppose we have a new food additive occurring as a 25% sodium salt and the proposed use will lead to the consumption of 1 g/day or about 15 mg/kg. The sodium requirement of the pregnant rat is 100 mg/day and most natural or purified diets furnish 300-400 mg of Na/Kg/day. Using 100 and 200-fold exaggerations in an animal study will lead to 375 and 750 mg of extra sodium/Kg or total sodium intakes of 675 and 1050 mg/kg. The acute oral LD50 of NaCl is about 4g/Kg., but on a chronic dietary basis 2-2.5% NaCl in a diet, equivalent to about 2g/Kg, will begin to produce toxicity as reflected in lower weight gains, diuresis, and glomerulitis. Since NaCl is less than half

TABLE 6   Representative Food Additives

Additive	Permitted Level in Foods ppm
BHA	2-200
Disodium EDTA	75-300
Sodium Lauryl Sulfate	125-1000
Potassium Nitrate	200
Sodium Nitrate	200

TABLE 7   Hypothetical Food Additive

Sodium Salt Food Additive = 25% Na
Food Additive Use   = 1 gm or 15 mg/Kg/Day

Diet Furnishes = 300 mg/Kg

100-Fold Exaggeration (100 x 15 x 25%) = 375 mg/Kg of Na
200-Fold Exaggeration (200 x 15 x 25%) = 750 mg/Kg of Na

Dietary Na + Test Na, Level #1 = 675 mg/Kg/day
Dietary Na + Test Na, Level #2 = 1050 mg/Kg/day

Oral LD_{50} of NaCl = 4 g/Kg
Threshold Toxicity of NaCl = 2 g/Kg or lg of Na/Kg/day

sodium, you can see that the high food additive test diet will probably produce some sodium toxicity and confound the experiment. Several control groups will be needed in a study of this material.

Similar situations can occur with other trace nutrients, but in addition to excesses one must beware of inducing deficiencies because of antagonisims or sequestering actions. Phytates sequestering zinc, that I mentioned earlier is a good example. Another, is that high levels of dietary fats, especially saturated ones, react with dietary calcium forming soaps, which decreases the intestinal absorption of both. Excessive phosphates may alter the Ca/P ratio to such an extent that either fetal bone calcification or lactation or both may be affected.

These examples of problems and perturbations in nutritional or food safety studies are just a few, but they illustrate the problems with attempting to determine reproductive toxicity and teratogenic potential of food components, and food additives, as well as naturally occurring toxicants in foods. I've also attempted to show that the design of the dietary components is probably the most important element of the overall design of the study. It is very important that all elements in the diet be as balanced as possible across control and test groups. Because of some of the factors I've discussed, other elements in the experimental design may need to be different than the usual toxicological study.

First, several control groups may be needed rather than the usual one or two. In the sodium salt example that I used, several control groups may be needed to establish the effects of the excess sodium versus those that may be caused by the sodium salt-food additive. Where nutritional extremes cannot be avoided, and many times they can't, then the appropriate controls must be carefully selected.

For most food materials, I prefer a reproductive study that combines Segments I, II and III of the FDA Guidelines (Figure 1, Table 8). This design allows a determination of the effects of the food material given chronically during the development of the parental reproductive systems, as well as on the current reproductive process. This includes effects on embryogenesis and fetal and neonatal development. The interpretation of teratogenic data is improved, since by now you know something of the overall reproductive capability of the animals within the variance framework of a single batch of contemporary animals.

Design of Reproduction-Teratology Study

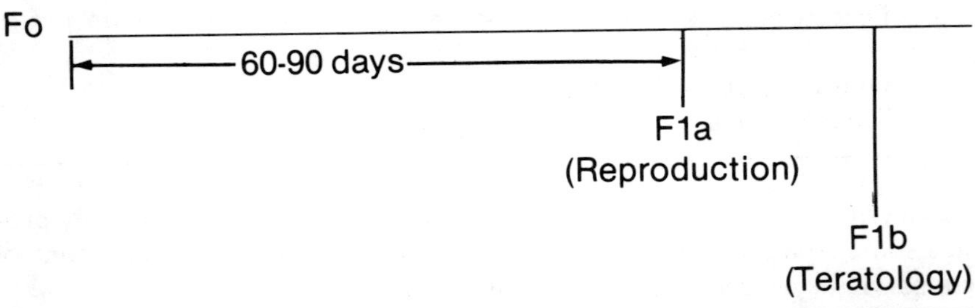

In this study, weanling rats are obtained and started immediately on the experimental regimen. Depending upon the material, eithr a single or multiple generation may be used. After 60-90 days, some of the rats are sacrificed and examined for histopathology, while the remaining ones are mated. The females are allowed to deliver and suckle their young. After weaning, the females are mated a second time, but this time they are sacrificed on day 20 of gestation and the usual teratologic parameters evaluated.

The interpretation of the data from studies such as these is fairly straight forward, as long as one keeps in mind the elements and interactions discussed here this morning, and as long as each study is designed carefully around the material under investigation. Changes in the test groups must be

TABLE 8

Time	Age of Rats	Action
Days	Days	
0	21- 23	Obtain From Supplier
7	28- 30	Start On Experiment
60- 90	90-120	Sacrifice Part - Histopath,
		Hematology, etc.,
70-110	100-130	Mate
91-131	121-151	Birth Of Fia
112-143	142-172	Wean Fia
122-153	152-182	Rest Dams
132-163	162-192	Mate
152-183	182-202	Sacrifice Dams on Day 20
		of Gestation

weighed very carefully against the various control groups, since changes in such things as fetal size, fetal developmental stages, or neonatal viability may well be due to secondary causes.

Although epidemiology studies and birth registries do not indicate that foods in general create significant reproductive hazards, nevertheless we know that such hazards can occur. Carefully designed animal studies can help establish the safety of new foods and food additives, but such studies demand some special attention. I have attempted to illustrate a few of these factors and situations.

REFERENCES

1. Hurley, L.S., Nutritional Deficiences and Excesses, IN: Handbook of Teratoplogy, Vol. I, pp. 287-289, Ed. J. G. Wilson and F. Clarke Fraser, Plenum Press, New York, 1977.
2. Nishimura, H., Chemistry and Prevention of Congenital Anomalies, pp. 31-32, Charles C. Thomas, Springfield, Ill, 1964.
3. Prasad, A. S., Halsted, J. A., and M. Nadimi, Syndrome of Iron Deficiency Anemia, Hepatosplenomegly, Hypogonadism, Dwarfism and Geophagia, Am. J. Med. *31,* 532-546, 1961.
4. Wilson, J. G., Environmental Chemicals, IN: Handbook of Teratology, Vol. I pp. 357-366, Ed. J. G. Wilson and F. Clarke Fraser, Plenum Press, New York, 1977.
5. Swenerton, H. and L. S. Hurley, Teratogenic Effects of a Chelating Agent and Their Prevention by Zinc. Science *173* 62-64, 1971.
6. Food Chemical News, p. 50, March 31, 1980.
7. Holson, J. F., Gaylor, D.W. Schumacher, H. J., Collins, T. F. X.,

Ruggles, D. I., Keplinger, W. L. annd G. L. Kennedy, Jr., Teratological Evaluation of FD&C Red No. 2 - A Collaborative Government - Industry Study. V. Combined Findings and Discussion. J. Toxicol. & Environ. Health *1*, 875-885, 1976.

8. Singh, A. R., Lawrence, W. H. and J. Autian, Teratogenicity of Phthalate Esters in Rats. J. Pharm. Sci. *61*, 51-55, 1972.

9. Boyd, E. M., Toxicity of Pure Foods, Ed. Carl E. Boyd, p. 71-111 CRC Press, Cleveland, Ohio, 1973.

10. Report of the American Institute of Nutrition Ad Hoc Committee on Standards for Nutritional Studies. J. Nutr. *107*, 1340-1348, 1977.

11. Warner, R.L., Nutrient Requirements of the Laboratory Rat, Nutrient Requirements of Domestic Animals No. 10, National Research Council, 1972.

12. Harper, A. E., Amino Acids of Nutritional Importance, IN: Toxicants Occurring Naturally in Foods, 2nd Ed., Committee on Food Protection, National Academy of Sciences, 1973.

CHAPTER 5

PETROLEUM AND PETROLEUM PRODUCTS: A BRIEF REVIEW OF STUDIES TO EVALUATE REPRODUCTIVE EFFECTS

C.A. Schreiner, Ph.D.
Environmental and Health Science Laboratory
Mobil Oil Corporation
P.O. Box 1026
Princeton, New Jersey 08540

SUMMARY

This article describes the types of studies being performed in the laboratory and in the field to identify reproductive effects of petroleum and petrochemicals. It includes discussions on the teratogenic risk from benzene, styrene and acrylonitrile, as representative petrochemicals. The extensive testing sponsored and overseen by the American Petroleum Institute to determine risk from workplace exposure to petroleum products is outlined. Wildlife studies which assess the effects of oil spills on waterfowl, fish and invertebrates are also presented.

INTRODUCTION

The information presented here, reviews some of the research being performed to identify reproductive risks from petroleum and petroleum products. Petroleum products are involved in most facets of modern life. They include fuels, lubricants and industrial solvents. According to Hawley's Chemical Dictionary, a petrochemical is an organic compound for which petroleum or natural gas is the ultimate material. This covers a multitude of compounds, including paraffins, olefins, aromatic hydrocarbons such as benzene, toluene, ethylene and plastics. Ethylene glycol can be considered a petrochemical because petroleum cracking produces ethylene. Synthetic fertilizers can also be petrochemicals.

The populations exposed to petroleum and petroleum products are varied. They include the human population through both workplace and environmental exposure, domestic animals and wildlife populations. Seabirds, fish and aquatic invertebrates are particularly at risk from oil spills.

TABLE 1

BENZENE TERATOLOGY AND RELATED STUDIES

STUDY	SPECIES	EXPOSURE LEVEL	ROUTE AND DURATION OF EXPOSURE	DECREASED MATERNAL WEIGHT GAIN	DECREASED FETAL WEIGHT GAIN	COMMENTS OR OBSERVATIONS
Watanabe & Yoshida (1970)	Mouse	3 ml/kg	Subcutaneous Single dose Day 11-15 of gestation	None	---	Day 13- Cleft palate, agnathia, micrognathia
Lyon (1975)	Rat	0.5 ml/kg	Intraperitoneal Acute dose - Male premating	Not Applicable	---	No effect from exposure of male in Dominant Lethal Study
Nawrot & Staples (1979)	Mouse	0.3-1.0 ml/kg (3 x/day)	Gavage - Daily Day 6-15; 12-15 of gestation		Yes	Embryonic resorption, Maternal lethality

From : Mehlman et al. 1980

Petrochemicals: Benzene, styrene and acrylonitrite were selected as representative petrochemicals based on widespread usage.

Benzene is one of the most extensively tested solvents. The degree of reproductive risk associated with benzene exposure is actively debated. The pancytopenia seen in workers exposed to benzene has led to concern that the solvent could adversely affect germ cells. Forni, et al. (1) and Picciano (2) correlated industrial exposure to benzene with chromosome damage and other abberations in blood cells. Hett and Maak (3) and Vara and Kinnuen (4) exposed female mice and rabbits respectively, to sufficient benzene to induce blood dyscrasias and observed degeneration of ovarian follicles and chromosome damage.

The first report of benzene induced teratogenicity was by Watanabe and Yoshida (5) who introduced a very high single dose (3 ml/kg) of benzene subcutaneously to pregnant mice on either day 11, 12, 13, 14, or 15 gestation (Table 1). Only fetuses exposed on day 13 were sensitive, demonstrating cleft palate, agnathia, micrognathia. However, Nawrot and Staples (6) induced increased resorption, but no malformation with a total oral daily doseof 3 ml/kg (1 ml/kg/t.i.d.) through embryogenesis in the rat. Lyon (7) reported no reproductive effect from a single dose of 0.5 ml/kg intraperitoneally to male rats prior to mating.

Since humans are exposed to benzene primarily via inhalation, the next two tables summarize studies using this route of exposure. Decreased litter size and decreased fetal weight gain were the major observations when benzene was administered to rats daily prior to and throughout pregnancy at doses from 6.3 to 560 ppm (Table 2). There were no malformations.

When benzene inhalation exposure was limited to the period of organogenesis in rats, mice and rabbits at doses 10-2200 ppm sufficient to induce maternal and fetal weight effects, few developmental anomalies were observed (Table 3). Increased resorptions were reported in one study at unexpectedly low doses.

Thus, exposure to benzene orally or parenterally at concentrations which induce overt maternal toxicity has caused embryo lethality, reduced fetal weight and in some instances malformations. Chronic inhalation of benzene resulted in only slight skeletal variations. The conceptus does not appear to be uniquely susceptible to benzene; rather, effects on development occur only at doses which produce maternal toxicity – Benzene is a "co-affective teratogen" as defined by E.M. Johnson. (8)

TABLE 2   REVIEW OF BENZENE INHALATION TERATOLOGY STUDIES

STUDY	SPECIES	EXPOSURE LEVEL	ROUTE AND DURATION OF EXPOSURE	DECREASED MATERNAL WEIGHT GAIN	DECREASED FETAL WEIGHT GAIN	COMMENTS OR OBSERVATIONS
Gofmekler (1968)	Rat	6.3-210 ppm	Inhalation 24 Hr/Day 10-15 days prior to impregnation	-	-	Decreased litter size
Pushkina et al. (1968)	Rat	1-670 mg/m^3 (208 ppm)	Inhalation throughout pregnancy	-	-	Decreased size size
Vozovaya (1975)	Rat	1783 mg/m^3 (559 ppm)	Inhalation 4 mo prior plus pregnancy	-	Yes - not sig.	No malformations for two generations
Vozovaya (1976)	Rat	370 mg/m^3 (116 ppm)	"	-	Yes	No malformations
Hudak & Ungvary (1978)	Rat Mouse	1000 mg/m^3 (310 ppm)	Inhalation 24 Hr/Day 1 to 14 days of pregnancy	-	Yes	No malformations

From: Mehlman et al. 1980

TABLE 3   SUMMARY OF BENZENE INHALATION TERATOLOGY

CONTRACTOR	SPECIES	STRAIN	INHALATION EXPOSURE LEVEL (PPM)	DURATION	DECREASED MATERNAL BODY WEIGHT	DECREASED FETAL BODY WEIGHT	DECREASED CROWN-RUMP DISTANCE	COMMENTS OR OBSERVATIONS
Hazleton 1977	Rat	Sprague-Dawley	0	day 6-	-	-	-	-
			10	day 16	-	-	-	-
			50	of	Yes*	Yes*	-	-
			500	gestation	Yes*	Yes*	Yes*	malformations[1]
Green et al. 1978	Rat	Sprague-Dawley	100	day 6-	-	-	-	missing sternebrae* (most in females)
			300	day 16 of	-	-	-	
			2,200	gestation	Yes*	Yes*	Yes*	missing sternebrae* (most in females)
Murray et al. 1979	Mouse	CF-1	500	day 6- day 15 of gestation	-	Yes*	-	missing sternebrae delayed skull ossi-fication; unfused occipital
	Rabbit	New Zealand	500	day 6- day 18 of gestation	-	-	-	extra ribs[2]; lum-bar spur(s); fused ribs, fused thoracic vertebrae (1 pup each/2 litters) gastroschisis (1 pup)
Litton Bionetics 1978	Rat	COBS^{TM} - Sprague Dawley	10	day 6-	-	-	-	increased resorptions
			40	day 16 of gestation	-	-	-	increased resorptions

* Statistically significant (p<0.05)

(1) Exencephaly, angulated ribs, non-sequential ossification of forefeet   (2) Occurred less often in litters of rabbits exposed to benzene

From: Mehlman *et al.* 1980

TABLE 4

STYRENE TERATOLOGY

STUDY	SPECIES	COMPOUND	EXPOSURE	ROUTE AND DURATION OF EXPOSURE	MATERNAL EFFECTS	FETAL EFFECTS	OBSERVATIONS
Murray *et al.* 1978	Rabbit	Styrene	300 ppm 600 ppm	Inhalation- 7 hrs/day day 6-18 of gestation	none	none	none unossified 5th sternabrae
	Rat	Styrene	300 ppm 600 ppm	Inhalation- 7 hrs/day day 6-15 of gestation	1 death dec. wt. gain days 6-9	dec. crown- rump length none	lumber spurs delayed ossification of sternebrae and vertebral centra
	Rat	Styrene	300 mg/kg	Gavage-daily day 6-15 of gestation	dec. weight gain days 6-9	none	renal agenesis- (1 pup/litter) at each dose
Ragule 1974	Rat	Styrene	0.35, 1.2, 12 ppm	Inhalation 4 hr/day throughout gestation		Increased resorptions	none reported
Vainio *et al.* 1977	Chick Embryo	Styrene	2-100 μmol/ egg	Injection into air space day 1-9 of development		LD_{50} 40μmol stunted growth	cyclopia, deformities of eyelid, bill, skull, lower extremities, brain hemorrhage,
		Styrene Oxide	0.5-5.0 μmol/egg			LD_{50} 1.5μmol	exencephaly

TABLE 5

ACRYLONITRILE TERATOLOGY

STUDY	SPECIES	EXPOSURE	ROUTE AND DURATION OF EXPOSURE	MATERNAL EFFECTS	FETAL EFECTS	OBSERVATIONS[a]
Murray *et al.* 1978	Rat	10 mg/kg	Gavage - daily day 6-15 of gestation	-		-
		25 mg/kg		-		short tail, short trunk missing vertebrae right-sided aortic arch
		65 mg/kg		1 death hyperexcitable excess salivation dec. pregnancies dec. wt gain gastric thickening	dec. body wt. dec. crown-rump length	
		40 ppm	Inhalation 6 hr/day	dec. wt gain	none	-
		80 ppm	day 6-15 of gestation	dec wt gain		short tail, short trunk, missing vertebrae, omphalocele hemivertebra

[a] Malformations statistically significant (P=0.05) at 65 mg/kg dosage only.

Styrene monomer is used in the manufacture of plastic, synthetic rubber, latex and resins (Table 4). Stewart *et al.* (9) reported transient neurological impairment, eye and nasal irritation in humans exposed to 376 ppm for up to 7 hours. Vainio *et al.* (10) screening styrene and styrene oxide in chick embryos reported a variety of malformations. Embryos exposed on day 0 and 1 of incubation were most vulnerable to lethality and teratogenic effects. Ragule (11) exposed rats throughout gestation to styrene by inhalation, resulting in increased resorptions at all dose levels, but no malformation. However, there were no resorptions among Ragule's control population, an unusual occurance. When Murray *et al.* (12) exposed rats and rabbits to styrene inhalation during organogenesis and an additional group of rats to styrene by gavage, no statistically significant incidence of fetal malformations was reported and no increase in resorptions was observed. Styrene may, as benzene, prove to be a co-affective teratogen.

Acrylonitrile, copolymerized with other monomers, is widely used in the production of various plastics and fibers (Table 5). It has demonstrated toxicity in the central nervous system, gastro-intestinal tract, respiratory tract and peripheral blood. Murray *et al.* (32) tested acrylonitrile in rats by gavage, because of human exposure via trace amounts of polymer migration into food from containers, and by inhalation, as the route of exposure in the workplace. An oral dose of 65 mg/kg/day was maternally toxic, decreased the pregnancy ratio and induced fetal malformations in 4% of the fetuses (8/212) from 35% litters (6/17) examined. Inhalation exposure caused decreased maternal weight gain at both levels. At 80 ppm malformations were observed, but the incidence was not significant. These data suggest that acrylonitrile may interfere with embryonal and fetal development at doses which are not maternally toxic, but additional studies are needed to verify the results.

API STUDIES

The American Petroleum Institute provides a coordinating center for cooperative research in the petroleum industry. Teratology studies are performed on chemically characterized API standard materials—fuels, oils and their components—representative of industry-wide formulations.

The purpose of these studies is to identify teratogenic risk at potential levels of workplace exposure rather than at massive doses used to evaluate intrinsic teratogenic effects (Table 6). Materials are administered to rats by inhalation, the most likely route of industrial human exposure. Dosage levels include the threshold limit value (TLV) previously established in toxicity studies and four times the TLV. Animals are exposed 6 hours daily from day 6-15 of gestation and sacrificed on day 20.

Table 6 summarizes the most recently completed API studies on fuels, solvents and petrochemicals. As one can see, rat fetuses do not appear to be particularly vulnerable to these oil products via maternal inhalation. Ongoing and proposed studies include testing of lubricating oils, new and used transmission fluids, additional heating fuel, gasoline and diesel fuel formulations as well as solvents and petrochemicals. It is a prodigious task, so if some rapid prescreen could be developed to prioritize these compounds for mammalian testing, it would be extremely useful.

TABLE 6

AMERICAN PETROLEUM INSTITUTE

INHALATION TERATOLOGY STUDIES - RAT

	Test Material	Dosage (ppm)	Results	
Fuels:	Unleaded Gasoline	400, 1600	Negative	
	Jet Fuel A	100, 400	Negative	
	Kerosene	100, 365	Negative	
	Diesel Fuel	100, 400	Negative	decrease maternal food consumption at 400 ppm
	Fuel Oil #2	85, 410	Negative	
Solvents:	Naphtha	100, 400	Negative	
	Stoddard Solvent	100, 400	Negative	
	70 Solvent	100, 400	Negative	
Petro Chemicals:	Benzene	10-500	Negative	decrease maternal and fetal body weights at 50, 500 ppm
	Toluene	100, 400	Negative	
	Xylene	100, 400	Negative	
	n-hexane	100, 400	Negative	
Shale:	Raw Dust	25-100 mg/m^3	Negative	
	Retorted	25-100 mg/m^3	Negative	
	Shale Oil	5-100 mg/m^3	Negative	embryotoxic at 100 mg/m^3 (RO-3)

WILDLIFE STUDIES

In the initial literature review, I found that a variety of interesting work has been done on the potential effects of oil spills on wildlife, particularly in reference to sea birds. Persistent spillage of petroleum over the past 50 years has become a major factor contributing to the decline of many colonies of sea birds. Much of the work described was done at the Patuxent Wildlife Research Center in Laurel, Md. Most of the crude and refined petroleum evaluated are reference samples supplied by, and characterized by API.

Table 7 summarizes three studies in which birds were treated orally with crude and refined petroleum. Ingestion of petroleum in sufficient quantities can result in decreased egg production, delayed onset of laying, reduced shell thickness, decreased fertilization and decreased hatchability. Engel *et al.* (13) reported that in Japanese quail the direct effect of crude oil was a decline in egg production at 800 mg but the concomitant fasting caused reduced egg weight and reduced shell thickness. Holmes *et al.* (14) in an earlier study noted that mallard ducks reared on a diet contaminated with South Louisiana crude oil did not mature sexually as efficiently as untreated birds and failed to display characteristic courtship behavior as frequently. All these effects of petroleum exposure were reversible. Where single doses were administered, normal reproductive patterns were re-established three days after dosage. When mallards ingesting 1 or 3 ml of South Louisiana crude oil for 150 days were returned to normal diets, normal rates of ovo-position, fertilization and hatchability were re-established within 5 days. The South Louisiana crude and Kuwait crude oil affected mallard reproduction differently - South Louisiana crude impairing spermatogenesis and storage and viability of sperm in female because fertilization is affected, Kuwait crude at high doses altering vitellogenesis and differentiation of ovarian follicles causing cessation of oviposition, - demonstrating that oils from different areas of the world differing in metal content and aromatic hydrocarbon concentration affect different stages of reproduction.

Miller *et al.* (15) demonstrated that ingestion of petroleum by herring gulls was followed by increase in mixed function oxidase activity and enhanced metabolism of corticosteroids. In mammals, impaired ovarian function is associated with stress-induced increases in adrenocorticoid activity. Diminished reproduction in birds may be in response to prolonged stress and high levels of corticotropin. Since marine birds normally sustain high levels of adrenocortical activity to maintain osmotic balance, additional stress may make them particularly vulnerable. (14)

Table 8 summarizes studies in which oil was applied to the surface of fertile eggs at various stages of incubation. Although birds themselves may not be heavily coated with oil following a spill, oil adhering to feathers and feet of breeding birds can be transferred to eggs, reducing hatchability. Significant effects on viability and embryo size have been demonstrated when as little as 1 μl is applied to the egg surface just below the air space. Previously, oil embryotoxicity was often attributed to blockage of pores on egg shell surface and

TABLE 7

INGESTION OF PETROLEUM BY WILD FOWL

STUDY	TEST MATERIAL	SPECIES	ROUTE OF INGESTION	DOSAGE	OBSERVATIONS
Engel *et al.* 1978	Prudhoe Bay Crude Oil	Japanese Quail F	Oral- Capsule Single Dose	400 mg/bird	decreased food consumption thin shell, decreased egg weight
				800 mg/bird	decreased food consumption thin shell, decreased egg weight, decreased egg production
Grau *et al.* 1977	Bunker C Oil	Japanese Quail F	Oral - Capsule Single Dose	200 mg/bird	decreased egg production reduced hatchability
Holmes *et al.* 1978	Southern Louisiana Crude Oil Kuwait Crude Oil	Mallard Ducks M, F	diet	1 ml/100 g diet	none
			150-200 days	3 ml/100 g diet	atretic ovaries decreased oviposition delay in laying onset decreased fertilization reduced hatchability thin shell (Louisiana crude)

TABLE 8   EFFECTS OF PETROLEUM EXPOSURE ON BIRD EGGS

STUDY	TEST MATERIAL	SPECIES	DOSAGE	OBSERVATIONS
Albers & Szaro 1978	No. 2 Fuel Oil	Common Eider	5, 20 μl single dose on shell surface, eggs returned to nest	20% decreased hatchability
Albers 1978	No. 2 Fuel Oil	Mallard Duck	5 μl single dose on shell surface 4 day intervals 26 day incubation	decreased hatchability – day 1-10 sensitive/deformed bills on dead embryos/South Louisiana crude > No. 2 Fuel Oil
Hoffman 1978	South Louisiana Crude Oil	Mallard Duck	5 μl paraffin 1, 5 μl oil day 3 incubation	no effect decreased hatchability at 5 μl day 4-6 (40%) 8-10 (51%) decreased body and bill length 66.7% abnormal survivors
	paraffin	White Leghorn Chick	5 μl paraffin 1, 5, μl oil day 2 incubation	no effect decreased hatchability at 5 μl day 7-9 (70%) decreased body and beak length 79.5% abnormal survivors
Hoffman 1979	South Louisiana Crude Oil	Mallard Duck	1, 5, 10 μl day 1 of incubation	decreased hatchability decreased body and bill length deformed bills; incomplete ossification reduced liver lobes incomplete feather formation stunting

interference with oxygen supply. This theory is refuted by the fact that a quantity of oil incapable of covering more than 5% of the shell surface is toxic and the fact that testing of the paraffinic portion most likely to block pores (16, 17) is not toxic. Albers (18) reported that hatchability decreases as the age of the embryo at treatment decreases. This was confirmed by Hoffman (17, 19), who also showed that exposure at day 1 of incubation not only caused extensive mortality, but increased the incidence of malformations among survivors. Malformations include deformed bills, incomplete ossification of skulls and stunting with incomplete feather formation. Hoffman postulates that the bimodal decrease in hatchability seen in mallard ducks may be correlated with the prominence of the yolk sac or chorioallantoic membrane in embryonic development. The lethalities from days 4-6 may be attributable to sequestering of oil aromatic components in the lipid fraction of yolk of mallard eggs which has a higher lipid content than that of chicken eggs which show no increase in mortality at this time. Lethalities in both species over days 7-10 correlate with the rapid outgrowth of the chorio-allantoic membrane over the surface of the inner shell membrane, providing a highly vascularized network for the rapid uptake of oil by this membrane.

The two remaining tables list a few studies performed in other species to illustrate the variety of reproductive testing underway to evaluate the risks to living organisms of unintentional exposure to petroleum and petroleum products. Some fish eggs and larval stages are resistant to crude oil and water soluble and aromatic fractions of crude oil and water soluble and aromatic fractions of crude oil, probably due to metabolic conversion by detoxifying enzymes, followed by rapid depuration and physiological homeostasis. (20) However, effects are more severe at all life stages if fish are stressed by environmental factors or poor nutrition. Females at spawning are poorly fed and, for migratory species, are subjected to environmental stress. Using benzene as a representative monoaromatic component of petroleum, Struhsaker (21) demonstrated abnormal behavior, premature spawning and reduced offspring survival in the pacific herring (Table 9). Linden (22) demonstrated toxic effects of a light fuel oil and two North Sea crude oils on Baltic herring eggs and subsequent larvae. Exposure of the estuarine stickle back to the water-soluble fraction of No. 2 fuel oil caused early hatching.

Exposure of invertebrates to water soluble petroleum fractions under controlled laboratory conditions decreased reproductive efficiency and offspring survival (Table 10). Le Roux and Lucas (29) exposed mussels to water soluble fractions extracted from Amoco Cadiz crude oil recovered at shoreline 18 hours after the grounding. At concentrations one to two order of magnitude higher than the highest concentrations found in water most severely impacted by Amoco Cadiz oil,fertilization and embryonic development were inhibited. Donahue *et al.* (30), evaluating water soluble fractions of eight petroleum oils in separate experiments, demonstrated impaired development in barnacle eggs and larvae exposed to No. 2 crude oil or naphthalene.

Inhibitory effects are reversible either by dilution of petroleum fractions over succeeding generations or when larvae can be returned to hydrocarbon-free salt water as demonstrated by Rossi and Anderson (23).

TABLE 9

REPRODUCTION EFFECTS OF PETROLEUM EXPOSURE IN FISH

STUDY	TEST MATERIAL	SPECIES	DOSAGE	OBSERVATIONS
Struhasker 1977	Benzene	Pacific herring- Spawning M, F	100 ppb 800 ppb	premature spawning disequilibrium decreased survival: egs 25%, embryos 26%, hatchings 43%
Linden 1978	No. 1 Fuel Oil North Sea Crude Oil	Baltie herring eggs -	exposed 6, 72 hrs. post fertilization 3.1-8.9 ppm 5.3-11.9 ppm	decreased heart rate altered activity altered hatching time 70-100% malformed larvae hatched or died day 1 posthatch
Ernst *et al.* 1977	No. 2 Fuel Oil Water Soluble Fraction	Fundulus grandis	dilutions: 12.5% 25.0% 50%	early hatching pathology of liver, kidney, lens, epitheleum/100% mortality
Anderson *et al.* 1980	Oil Shale Process Water	Rainbow Trout Eggs	dilution: 0.16%	decreased hatchability decreased size

TABLE 10

REPRODUCTIVE EFFECTS OF PETROLEUM EXPOSURE IN INVERTEBRATES

STUDY	TEST MATERIAL	SPECIES	DOSAGE	OBSERVATIONS
Le Roux & Lucas 1978	Crude petroleum (Amoco Cadiz)	Mussel	10 ml/l sea H_2O	inhibited mussel egg fertilization, embryo development abnormal larvae
Donahue *et al.* 1977	Water soluble fractions of 8 petroleum oils	Barnacles - eggs larvae	3 ppm	decreased embryonic development and larval activity induced by No. 2 fuel oil, naphthalene
Rossi & Anderson 1978	No. 2 fuel oil	Neanthis arenaceodentata (Annelid)	dilution: 2.5% 5.0% 10.0% 25.0%	inhibit oocyte maturation decreased hatchability, maturation with increased exposure and concentration sensitivity: juveniles > larvae

Although the experiments described attempt to simulate in the laboratory the possible effects of petroleum exposure at sea or through continuous low level pollution of confined waters as in city harbors, it should be recognized that many additional factors determine biological effects on avian and aquatic populations. These factors include the size and range of the population, individual sensitivities, fecundity and mechanisms of detoxification. Laboratory studies identify intrinsic "worse case" effects, but are not definitive for risk estimation. While some studies monitor toxicity, others demonstrate reversibility. Continued development of rapid efficient and non-toxic methods of cleaning up oil spills can save a substantial percentage of an exposed population and future generations. Overall, laboratory tests should complement field studies in contributing to the understanding of petroleum effects on living organisms.

REFERENCES

1. Forni, A. Picifico E., Limonta, A., Arch. Environ. Health 22: 373-378, 1971.
2. Picciano, D., Environmental Research 19:33-38, 1979.
3. Hett, J., Mack, H., Klinische Wochenschrift 17:1376, 1938.
4. Vara, P., Kinnunen, O1. Act Obstet et Gynecol Scand26(3) 433-452, 1946.
5. Watanabe G., Yoshida, S., Acta. Medica et Biologia 17:285-291, 1970.
6. Nawrot, P.S., Staples, R.E., Teratol. 19(2):41A.
7. Lyon, J.P., Ph.D. thesis, University of California, 1975.
8. Johnson, E.M., Ann. Rev. Pharmacol, Toxicol. 21:417-429, 1981.
9. Stewart, R.D., Dobb, H.C., Baretta, E.D., Schaffer, A.W., Arch. Environ. Health 16:656, 1968.
10. Vanio, H., Hamminki, K., Elovaara, E. Toxicol. 8:319-325, 1977.
11. Ragule, N.Y., Gig. Sanit. 11:85-86, 1974.
12. Murray, F.J., John, J.A.,Balmer, M.F., Schwetz, B.A., Toxicol. 11:335-343, 1978.
13. Engel, S.E., Roudybush, T.E., Dobbs, J.C., Grau, C.R., DOE Symp. Ser., series 47, publ. 78:27-36, 1977.
14. Holmes, W.N., Cavanaugh, K.P., Cronshaw, J., J. Reprod. and Fert. 54:335-348, 1978.
15. Miller, D.S., Peakall, D.B., Kinter, W.B., Science 199:315-317, 1978.
16. Albers, P.H., Symposium on fate and effects of petroleum hydrocarbons in marine ecosystems and organisms. New York:Pergamon Press, pp. 158-163, 1977.
17. Hoffman, D.J., Toxicol. Appl. Pharmacol. 46:183-190, 1978.
18. Albers, P.G., Bull, Environ. Contam. Toxicol. 19:624-630, 1978.
19. Hoffman, D.J., Bull. Environ. Contam. Toxicol. 23:203-206, 1979.
20. Lee, R.F., Saverheber, R., Dobbs, G.H., Mar. Biol. 17:201-208, 1972.
21. Struhsaker, J.W., Fish Bull. 75:43-49, 1977.

22. Linden, O., Mar. Biol. 45:273-293, 1978.
23. Rossi, S.S., Anderson, J.W., Water, Air and Soil Pollut. 9:155-170, 1978.
24. Mehlman, M.A., Schreiner, C.A., Mackerer, C.R., J. Environ. Path. Toxicol. 4(5 & 6): 123-131, 1980.
25. American Petroleum Institute, Medicine and Biological Science Department Research Reports, 1979-1980.
26. Albers, P.H., Szaro, R.C., Marine Pollution Bulletin 9:138-139, 1978.
27. Ernst, *et al.*, Environ. Pollut. 14(1)25-26, 1977.
28. Anderson, A.D., Lebsack, M.E., Degrave, G.M., Farrier, D.S., Bergman, H.L., Arch. Environ. Contamin. Toxicol. 9:171-179, 1980.
29. LeRoux, S., Lucas, A., Publ. Cent. Nat. Exploit, Oceans 6:215-225, 1978.
30. Donahue, *et al.*, Environ. Pollut. 13:187-202, 1977.
31. Grau, C.R., Roudybush, T., Dobbs, J., Wathen, J., Science 195:779-781, 1977.
32. Murray, F.J., Schwetz, B.A., Nitschke, K.D., John, J.A., Norris, J.M., Gehring, P.J., Fd. Cosmet. Toxicol. 16: 547-551, 1978.

CHAPTER 6

REPRODUCTIVE TOXICOLOGY: RADIATION EFFECTS

Ronald P. Jensh, Ph.D.
Jefferson Medical College
Phila., Pa. 19107

Radiobiologic studies have been conducted for over half a century. Laws governing the use of radiation sources are much more restrictive than those governing the majority of other potentially hazardous products. Our knowledge in this highly complex area is extensive, but there are still many unanswered questions.

In order to understand radiation we must first define some terms. Radiation sources may be divided into 2 groups; those sources which are particulate and those which are produced by electromagnetic fields. Particulate radiation includes alpha particles, which are helium nuclei (2 protons and 2 neutrons), and beta particles, which are electrons which have been ejected from nuclei of unstable atoms. Other particles include neutrons, pions, and muons (15). To describe the other radiation source we must first understand the electromagnetic spectrum (see Table 1). Gamma- and x-rays originate from different sources. Gamma radiation originates from atomic nuclei. X-rays originate from outside the nuclei as high energy electrons are deflected from a target (15;19). The difference is in the origin rather than in the nature of the radiation. Gamma- and x-rays are ionizing because their photons have enough energy to cause ionization of molecules. Ionization is the process by which an electron is dislodged from its orbit. Ionization may occur as the result of the repulsive force occurring from an electron (beta) passing near to that orbital electron, by the attractive force of a positively charged particle (alpha), or may be due to an increased energy state being imparted to that electron (x-rays) (15). Alpha and beta particles are ionizing due to their high energy levels. Microwave radiation, however, is substantially lower in energy levels and, therefore, is non-ionizing. Microwave energy levels are in the area of 10-7 to 10-3 electron-volts.

In order to compare and contrast the effects of various forms of radiation on biologic systems, units of measurement must be defined. Roentgen (R) applies only to electromagnetic radiation and is a measure of the

47

TABLE 1   ELECTROMAGNETIC SPECTRUM

FREQUENCY (Hz)	WAVELENGTH (cm.)	TYPE	OSCILLATING SOURCE
3×10^{21}	10^{-11}	Gamma	nuclear charges
3×10^{20}	10^{-10}		
3×10^{19}	10^{-9}	X-rays	atomic inner shell electrons
3×10^{18}	10^{-8}		
3×10^{17}	10^{-7}	UV	atomic outer shell electrons
3×10^{16}	10^{-6}		
3×10^{15}	10^{-5}		
3×10^{14}	10^{-4}	Visible Light	atomic outer shell electrons
3×10^{13}	10^{-3}		
3×10^{12}	10^{-2}	Infrared	molecular vibrations
3×10^{11}	10^{-1}(1mm)		molecular vibrations
3×10^{10}	10^{0}(1cm)	Microwaves	
3×10^{9}	10^{1}		Klystrons, magnetrons
3×10^{8}	10^{2}(1m)	Radio, short wave	electronic circuits
3×10^{6}	10^{4}	Radio, long wave	

(from: Casarett, 1968; Curnutte, 1980; Lambert, 1980)

physical field, not the effect of the field on matter. Particulate radiation, such as alpha and beta, is measured in terms of the intensity or flux of the radiation at a given point in space. RAD (Radiation-Absorbed-Dose) is a measurement of energy deposition per gram of irradiated tissue. RBE (Relative-Biologic-Effectiveness) is a factor by which the RAD is multiplied to account for differences in sensitivity and reactivity among various cells and tissues. The QF (Quality Factor) has been related primarily to x-rays. It is an empirical quantity which has replaced the RBE when considering hazard levels. This factor takes into account a number of physical properties of the radiation. REM (Roentgen-Equivalent-Man) is also called the Dose Equivalent. This unit of measure is the product of the dose in RAD, the QF, and any other additional modifying factors (19).

The radiation effects which will be discussed are referable primarily to x-rays (ionizing) and microwaves (non-ionizing). Radio-isotopes (radionuclides) and their effects on the developing organism will not be included, since the sources are not of concern within the context of the present discussion. Generally their effects would be similar, however these sources have not been as extensively studied as has x-irradiation. Their effects would be due primarily to internal exposure and would be modified by the radionuclide's chemical structure, type and energy of radiation, and by the target organs involved. Thus placental interaction, metabolic activity, and many other variables would have to be considered. Also, exposure of pregnant women to radio-isotopes is comparatively rare (7).

There are a number of review articles which describe in detail the effects of irradiation on the developing organism (7;8;27;30;60). From the multitude of experiments several generalizations can be made. The absorbed dose, dose rate, and stage of gestation at the time of exposure are the major determinants of radiation effects. Exposure to varying dosage levels of radiation produces a classic absorbed dose response curve. Altering the dose rate will cause a shift in the dose response curve. A fractionated dose is less likely to produce malformations than a single acute exposure to the same dose. It may be that fractionation results in "normality" by allowing sufficient time for recuperative mechanisms to be activated (7;9).

The effects of prenatal radiation on the developing organism are defined as the "Triad". One effect is lethality, which includes embryonic and fetal death as well as perinatal, neonatal, and adult death (33). Another effect is abnormality. The majority of studies have restricted this effect to gross or semi-gross organ-system lesions which can be observed at term with the naked eye or with the aid of a dissecting microscope. Most recently this term has been considerably expanded to include functional and physiologic alterations; prenatally, perinatally, and postnatally. The third possible effect is growth retardation, which may be confined to intra-uterine life or may continue into extra-uterine life and persist throughout the lifetime of the individual (10). Each of these effects has a dose response curve relationship and a minimal threshold exposure level. The severity of each is dependent upon the absorbed dose, dose rate, and developmental stage at the time of exposure. Assuming constancy of the first 2 variables, what effects are stage dependent? That is, which triad effects would be expected from exposure to a single given dose of x-rays at a given dose rate at various times during pregnancy? For simplicity, the present discussion is based upon a single 200 R dose administered at a constant dose rate to pregnant rodents, such as has been done by Russell and Russell (1954)(61).

    1. Exposure during the PREBLASTOCYST OR PREIMPLANTA-

TION STAGE generally results in an all or none phenomenon; that is, lethality or normality. Little or no growth retardation or teratogenesis occurs, although growth retardation can occur at any time after this period. Teratogenesis (teratogenic activity) in this instance refers to gross morphologic malformations. Prenatal death rate progressively decreases to normality as the time of exposure moves toward the later stages of pregnancy.

2. Exposure during the POSTIMPLANTATION-PREORGANOGENIC STAGE results in less lethality than the previous stage. A low level of malformations occur, as well as some growth retardation. (Significant growth retardation is seen at 15O R, a dose which also produces death, although no significant increase in the incidence of malformations.)

3. Exposure during the EARLY ORGANOGENIC STAGE results in the appearance of the full triad. Generally growth retardation is recuperable. Exposure during this stage results in the highest incidence of gross malformations, as previously defined. The highest neonatal death rate also occurs from exposure during this stage (7). This stage corresponds to 5.5-11 days (peak: 7.5-8.5) in mice; 8-12 days (peak: 8.5-9.5) in rats, and 12-50 days (peak: 12-22) in man (6;8). A general rule is that the incidences of growth retardation and malformations are maximum during the period of most active differentiation. Central nervous system cell rosette formation can be seen from exposure at this time (54). One hundred R yields a high incidence of malformations, death, and growth retardation, but doses as low as 50 R are also teratogenic. Rugh and Wohlfromm (1965)(59) claim to have observed a significantly increased death rate from exposures as low as 25 R. We do not know the lowest dose that will produce growth retardation, although it is certainly below 100 R and is likely to be less than 50 R.

4. Exposure during the EARLY FETAL STAGE results in a progressively decreasing sensitivity to the malforming effects of radiation, although late developing systems such as the central nervous system are still sensitive. Growth retardation generally is recuperable postnatally, although often not completely.

5. Exposure during the LATE FETAL STAGE does not generally result in massive alterations in development. Often the effects are at the cellular level, with cell depletion at high exposure levels (11;29). Few gross structural malformations have been observed, but few postnatal analyses have been completed. Subtle changes may occur during the fetal stage, especially in specific organs or areas in organs, such as the central nervous system. Effects would be related specifically to the time and dose. For example, Hicks, et al (1959)(31) exposed pregnant rats to a single acute 200 R dose on days 13 to 17 of gestation. The degree of cerebral cortical atrophy in the offspring varied with the day of exposure. Postnatally a variety of behavior and motor deficits have been observed (66;27;12;68;67) while histologically the neuronal patterns were altered (31;1;18;30). Other organs that have been shown to be affected include the thyroid, diaphragm, and testes (5); the results being dose and time dependent. An interesting

phenomenon is the species-specific differential sensitivity of males and females to the sterilizing effects of irradiation. This differential sensitivity may be due to differing developmental sequencing of ova and spermatozoa (7;60;14;25;3;26;50;35;41).

Since the 1950's investigators such as Wilson (1954), Rugh (1960); Rugh and Grupp (1960), Russell and Russell (1954), Hicks (1953), and Brent (1960)(69;54;58;61;29;5) have been actively studying the teratogenic effects of ionizing radiation, particularly x-irradiation. Most recently Mullenix (1975) and Tamaki, et al (1976)(49;64;63) have shown postnatal functional alterations due to exposure late in gestation. Martin (1977), Takeuchi (1976), Das (1977),(1978), Rugh (1973), and Norton (1979)(46;62;21;22;55;51) have shown central nervous system alterations postnatally due to prenatal exposure to dosages of 100 R to 400 R late in gestation in both rodents and primates. In most instances these effects have not manifested themselves until adulthood.

Growth retardation and central nervous system alterations are the primary effects of irradiation seen in man, with microcephaly being the most common organic lesion. These effects were seen as early as 1929 by Goldstein and Murphy where growth retardation always accompanied the malformation. Human embryos exposed to a protracted 250 R dose between 3 and 20 weeks of age were microcephalic, mentally retarded, or both. All were growth retarded (23). Hiroshima and Nagasaki studies revealed similar results. There was some variation, however, probably due to the differing types of radiation produced (4;48;71;70). In fact, no radiation-induced morphological malformations have been reported in man without associated growth retardation or central nervous system abnormalities (7;9).

The human central nervous system is also radiosensitive in postnatal life, whereas other systems have a rather narrow age-range of sensitivity. Multiple system malformations result from prenatal exposure from 2 to 4 weeks in man and 9 to 13 days in rats. The percent of time of sensitivity is longer in the rat than in man considering the length of pregnancy. The patterns of cellular sensitivity, however, are similar in man and other mammals. This is most likely due to the fact that radiation effects are directly on the embryo and not solely mediated through the placental or maternal systems (9;40).

Radiation effects may be immediate or greatly delayed. The immediate effects of irradiation are obvious and include cell, tissue, organ, or entire organism death, size decrease, and abnormality. Delayed effects are more subtle and may include generalized growth retardation, hypoplastic organs, neoplasia, decreased cell numbers, behavioral alterations, functional alterations, and life-span shortening.

Hypotheses have been made concerning the many mechanisms by which radiation-induced damage can occur. It is difficult to determine which one or combinations are primarily responsible at any particular stage of pregnancy. Representative areas include cell death, cytogenetic abnormalities, somatic mutations, mitotic delay, cell migratory alterations, and a variety of biochemical alterations (9).

The dangers of large doses of ionizing radiation are obvious. There is much less agreement concerning low dose levels. The preimplantation stage LD 50 exposure level is less than 100 R. This dose level rises during implantation, falls during organogenesis, then rises to approach adult levels during the fetal stages. There is no stage at which 50 R is not associated with some embryopathic effect. Some growth retardation is always evident from irradiation levels greater than 100 R at any time after implantation. In man, absorption of more than 50 RAD at any time during pregnancy will result in a significant increase in risk of damage, especially to the central nervous system (9). If exposure occurs early in organogenesis the offspring may exhibit intrauterine growth retardation, but such growth effects may be recuperable postnatally. Exposure during the early fetal period will usually result in permanent growth retardation (7). At levels of several hundred RAD, especially early in pregnancy, abortion is the invariable result. The area of 10-20 RAD remains argumentative. Certainly dosages less than 5 RAD can be considered to be "no triad effect" levels (7;9). A practical threshold level has been considered to be 10 RAD since absorption of less than 10 RAD is not teratogenic as classically defined. The N.C.R.P. has recommended that the maximum permissible fetal dose throughout pregnancy should be 0.5 REM (7;52).

Diagnostic radiology is in the range of 20-5, 000 mRAD, which is a very low risk level. Five RAD is considered to be a no effect level based on the triad concept, but there may be other unknown subtle effects. Therefore, elective radiologic procedures should be limited to the first 14 days of the menstrual cycle. A pregnancy test might be a false negative even if the female waits 3 weeks, but the embryo would be entering the organogenic phase at 3 weeks and would be highly sensitive to radiation. Therefore, both the mother and child would be at risk. As Brent (1967)(10) has pointed out, "to procrastinate is to jeopardize".

Russell and Russell (1954)(61) presented a graphic summary of mouse data. Their results are still valid with a few modifications which have been discussed by Brent (1969)(6) and include: a. The fetus is not totally insensitive to teratogenesis, especially when considering the postnatal studies that have been previously discussed. b. Non-dysjunction of chromosomes can occur from exposure on the first day. c. The zygote is radiosensitive, but the degree of sensitivity depends on the phase of the cell cycle at the time of exposure. d. Low dosage level effects are seen throughout gestation. e. The mouse as a species has 2 unique idiosyncratic reactions; exencephaly and whole litter resorption.

The effects of microwave radiation on the developing organism have not been extensively studied. Biologic effects are frequency dependent since biologic molecules in general are highly polar. The biophysical properties of microwaves are quite unique and accurate dosimetry is still very difficult to perform (53).

The Federal Communications Commission (F.C.C.) has allotted specific frequencies of microwaves for commercial and domestic use. Therefore, these are the frequencies of greatest concern to man. Most biologic studies have been done at these frequencies. Specifically, the F.C.C. has assigned 4 microwave frequencies for use in the industrial, scientific, and medical fields. The 915 MHz and 2450 MHz frequencies are used for domestic and commercial food preparation and the 5800 MHz and 22,125 MHz frequencies are used for laboratory and research applications (44).

Almost all previous studies have been done in rodents at 2450 MHz. The teratogenic studies have been at power levels which have created a hyperthermic condition in the animal model. The primary mechanism of damage appears to be thermal, but there is no conclusive proof that the non-thermal effects do not exist (32;16;17;45). Rugh, et al (1975)(57) has observed teratogenic effects in mice resulting from exposure to 2450 MHz, but the power levels used would result in increased animal body temperature. His results are typical of those seen using a variety of techniques which raise the body temperature (57;56). Currently the threshold limit has been set at 10 mW/cm² for the frequency range of 300 MHz to 300 GHz (OSHA, 1971)(44).

A variety of mechanisms may be involved in the production of microwave effects on biologic systems. How these may relate to teratogenic activity is still unknown. Table 2 summarizes the types of biological effects which have been observed at various frequencies. A number of interactive mechanisms have also been postulated by Lambert (1980) (44), involving both "thermal" and "non-thermal" radiation levels.

Our laboratory has investigated the effects of microwave radiation throughout pregnancy at exposure levels which approach but do not cause an increase in body temperature. We have observed mothers and offspring exposed to 915 MHz, 2450 MHz, and 6000 MHz. Standard teratologic analyses as well as postnatal behavioral and functional analyses have been completed on several hundred exposed animals. No significant alterations have been noted in the studies at the 2 lower frequencies (32;34;38;39;43). Several interesting and provocative alterations occurred in the 6 GHz study. Subtle alterations in the onset of specific reflexes in the exposed offspring and growth retardation, and a small but significant increase in resorption rate in the second non-exposed generation were observed (42;36). If these results are confirmed, the implications could be wide-reaching since this frequency is used for telecommunications. The power levels are much higher than those to which the general population are exposed however. There are also specific species susceptibility differences which are frequency dependent (44); a variable which is not a factor in exposure to ionizing radiation.

Microwave teratologic research is highly controversial and will remain so until additional well-designed investigations are completed. Future studies will need to combine well controlled dosimetry with competent teratologic studies including subtle postnatal physiologic and functional evaluations.

TABLE 2   Thermal-Biological Effects of Microwaves

FREQUENCY (MHz)	WAVELENGTH	SITE, MAJOR TISSUE EFFECTS	MAJOR BIOLOGICAL EFFECTS
>10,000	<3	skin	skin absorbs/reflects with heating effects
10,000	3	skin	skin heating; feel warmth
10,000-3,300	3 to 10	top layers, skin; lens of eye	lens, testes very susceptible
10,000-1,000	3-30	lens	critical band for cataracts; gonad damage
1,200-150	25 to 200	internal organs	damage internally by overheating
<150	above 200		body transparent to wavelengths 200 cm.

(from: Environmental Health Services, 1969)

A great deal is known about the effects of ionizing radiation on the developing organism. Much less is understood concerning the action and inter-action of non-ionizing radiation on the prenatal, paternal, and maternal organism.

In order to achieve a better understanding of the effects of radiation exposure on human life, we must investigate further:

1.   the mechanisms of normal cell growth, replication, and differentiation in the timed sequence of embryonic and fetal development;

2.   the etiologies and associated mechanisms involved in abnormal growth and development;

3.   the mechanisms of action of the various forms of ionizing and non-ionizing radiations, including continued expansion of biophysical and physicochemical information;

4.   the interaction of all applicable forms of radiation with the living and growing organism, including prenatal and postnatal evaluations;

5.   the concept of dose rate as related to threshold levels;

6.   radiation threshold levels in general, in order to continue to refine our determinations of safety levels for the human population and to assure continued safe environment for the growth and development of succeeding generations.

REFERENCES

1. Altman, W.J., Anderson, W., and Wright, K. 1968. Reconstitution of the external granular layer of the cerebellar cortex in infant rats after low-level x-irradiation. Anat. Rec., 163:453.

2. Anderson, E.J., and Altman, J. 1972. Retardation of cerebellar and motor development in rats by focal x-irradiation beginning at four days. Physiol. Behavior., 8:57.

3. Beaumont, H. 1962. Effect of irradiation during fetal life on the subsequent structure and secretory activity of the gonads. J. Endocrinol., 24:325.

4. Blot, W., 1957. Growth and development following prenatal and childhood exposure to atomic radiation. J. Rad. Res., 16, Suppl.:82.

5. Brent, R.L. 1960. The effect of irradiation on the mammalian fetus. Clin. Obstet. Gynecol., 3:928.

6. Brent, R.L. 1969. The direct and indirect effects of irradiation upon the mammalian zygote, embryo and fetus. In: Nishimura, H., Miller, J.R., and Yasuda, M. (eds.), Methods for teratological studies in experimental animals and man: Proceedings of the second international workshop in teratology, Kyoto, Japan. Igaku Shin, Ltd., Tokyo, p. 63.

7. Brent, R.L. 1976. Environmental factors: Radiation. Chapter 9. In: Brent, R.L. and Harris, M.I. (eds.) Prevention of embryonic fetal and perinatal disease. N.I.H., DHEW Publication No. (NIH) 76-853, Bethesda, Md., p. 179.

8. Brent, R.L. 1977. Radiations and other physical agents. In: Wilson, J.G. and Fraser, F.C. (eds.), Handbook of teratology, Plenum Press, N.Y.C., p. 153.

9. Brent, R.L. 1980. Radiation teratogenesis. Teratol., 21:281.

10. Brent, R.L., and Jensh, R.P. 1967. Intrauterine growth retardation. In: Woollam, D.H.M. (ed.), Advances in teratology, volume 2, p. 139.

11. Brizzee, K.R., Jacobs, L.A., and Bench, C.J. 1967. Histologic effect of total body x-irradiation on various dose fractionation patterns on fetal cerebral hemisphere. Rad. Res., 31:415.

12. Brizzee, K.R., Jacobs, L., and Kharetchko, X. 1961a. Effects of total body x-irradiation in utero on early postnatal changes in neuron volumetric relationships and packing density in cerebral cortex. Rad. Res., 14:96.

13. Brizzee, K.R., Jacobs, L., and Kharetchko, X. 1961b. Quantitative histologic and behavioral studies on the effects of fetal x-irradiation on developing cerebral cortex of white rats. in: Haky, T.J. and Snider, R.S., (eds.), Response of the nervous system to ionizing radiation, Academic Press, N.Y.C.

14. Brown, S. 1964. Effects of continuous low intensity radiation on successive generations of the albino rat. Genetics, 50:1101.

15. Casarett, A.P. 1968. Radiation biology. Prentice-Hall, Inc., Englewood Cliffs, N.J.

16. Chernovetz, M.E., Justesen, D.R., King, H.W., and Wagner, J.E. 1975. Teratology, survival and reversal learning after fetal irradiation of mice by 2450 MHz microwave energy. J. Microwave Power, 10:391.

17. Chernovetz, M.E., Justesen, D.R., and Oke, A.T. 1977. A teratological study of the rat: microwave and infrared radiations compared. Radio. Sci., 12:191.

18. Cowen, D., and Geller, L.M. 1960. Long term pathological effects of prenatal x-irradiation on the central nervous system of the rat. J. Neuropathol. Exp. Neurol., 19:488.

19. Crawford, D.J., and Leggett, R.W. 1980. Assessing risk of exposure to radioactivity. Am. Sci., 68:524.

20. Curnutte, B. 1980. Principles of microwave radiation. J. Food Protection, 43(8): 618.

21. Das, G.D. 1977. Experimental analysis of embryogenesis of cerebellum in the rat. II. Morphogenetic malformations following x-ray irradiation on day 18 of gestation. J. Comp. Neurol., 176(3):435.

22. Das, G.D. 1978. Premature death of purkinje cells following low-level x-ray irradiation during embryonic development. Acta Anat., 101:225.

23. Dekaban, A.S. 1968. Abnormalities in children exposed to x-irradiation during various stages of gestation: tentative timetable of

radiation injury to the human fetus. J. Nucl. Med., 9:471.
24. Environmental Health Series, USDHEW, 1969. Regulations, standards, and guide for microwave, ultraviolet radiation, and radiation from lasers and television receivers.
25. Ershoff, B., and Bratt, V. 1960. Comparative effects of prenatal gamma radiation and x-irradiation on the reproductive system of the rat. Am. J. Physiol., 198:1119.
26. Erikson, B., Murphree, R., and Andrews, J. 1963. Effects of prenatal gamma irradiation on the germ cells of the male pig. Rad. Res., 20:640.
27. Furchtgott, E. 1963. Behavioral effects of ionizing radiations: 1955-1961. Psychol. Bull., 60(2):157.
28. Goldstein, L., and Murphy, D.P. 1929. Microcephalic idiocy following radium therapy for uterine cancer during pregnancy. Am. J. Obstet. Gynecol., 18:189.
29. Hicks, S.P. 1953. Developmental malformations produced by radiation: A timetable of their development. Am.J. Roentgenol. Radium Therapy Nucl. Med., 69:272.
30. Hicks, S.P. and D'Amato, C.J. 1966. Effects of ionizing radiation of mammalian development. In: Woollam, D.H.M. (ed.), Advances in teratology, Logos Press, London, p. 196.
31. Hicks, S.P., D'Amato, C.J., and Lowe M.J. 1959. The development of the mammalian nervous system. I. Malformations of the brain, especially the cerebral cortex, induced in rats by radiation. J. Comp. Neurol., 113:435.
32. Jensh, R.P. 1980. Behavioural teratology: Application to low dose chronic microwave irradiation studies. In: Persaud, T.V.N. (ed.), Advances in the study of birth defects, Volume 4, Neural and behavioural teratology, International Medical Publishers, London, P. 135.
33. Jensh, R.P., Brent, R.L., and Bolden, B.T. 1969. The effect of prenatal x-irradiation on the length of postnatal life in mice. Teratol., 2:262.
34. Jensh, R.P., Brent, R.L., Ludlow, J., Weinberg, I., and Vogel, W.H. 1977. Teratologic effects on the rat offspring of non-thermal chronic prenatal microwave irradiation. Teratol., 15(2):14A.
35. Jensh, R.P., Garaguso, J.E., and Brent, R.L. 1973. The effects of prenatal x-irradiation on the reproductive performance of the male Wistar albino rat. Teratol., 7:18A.
36. Jensh, R.P., Ludlow, J., and McHugh T. 1980. Studies concerning the effects of protracted prenatal 6 GHz microwave irradiation on pre- and postnatal development in the rat. Teratol., 21(2):46A.
37. Jensh, R.P., Ludlow, J., Vogel, W.H., McHugh, T., Weinberg, I., and Brent, R.L. 1979a. Studies concerning the effects of non-thermal protracted prenatal 915 MHz microwave radiation on prenatal and postnatal develement in the rat. Digest of the XIV In-

ternational Microwave Symposium, Monaco, June 11-15 (IMPI), p. 99.

38. Jensh, R.P., Ludlow, J., Weinberg, I., Vogel, W.H., Rudder, T., and Brent, R.L. 1978a. Studies concerning the effects of protracted prenatal exposure to a non-thermal level of 2450 MHz microwave radiation on the pregnant rat. Teratol., 17(2):48A.

39. Jensh, R.P., Ludlow, J., Weinberg, I., Vogel, W.H., Rudder, T., and Brent, R.L. 1978b. Studies concerning the postnatal effects of protracted low dose prenatal 915 MHz microwave irradiation. Teratol., 17(2):21A.

40. Jensh, R.P., and Magalhaes, H. 1962. The effect of whole body x-irradiation on the central nervous system of golden hamster embryos. Proc. Pa. Acad. Sci., 36:194.

41. Jensh, R.P., Pugarelli, J.E., MacBain, S. and Brent, R.L. 1976. The effects of prenatal x-irradiation on the reproductive performance of Wistar albino rat. Teratol., 13:26A.

42. Jensh, R.P., Vogel, W.H., Ludlow, J., and McHugh, T. 1979b. Studies concerning the effects of low dosage prenatal 6000 MHz microwave radiation on growth and development in the rat. Teratol., 19(2):32A.

43. Jensh, R.P., Vogel, W.H., Ludlow, J., and McHugh, T. 1980b. Studies concerning the effects of non-thermal protracted 2450 MHz microwave irradiation on postnatal development in the rat. Teratol., 21(2):46A.

44. Lambert, J.P. 1980. Biological hazards of microwave radiation. J. Food Protection, 43(8):625.

45. Laskey, J., Dawes, D., and Howes, M. 1970. Progress report on 2450 MHz irradiation of pregnant rats and the effects on the fetus. In: Radiation Bio-effects Summary Report, Public Health Services, US DHEW/DRH/DBE-70, Rockville, Md., p. 167.

46. Martin, P.G. 1977. Response of the developing rat brain to varying doses and dose-rates of gamma radiation. Growth, 41:41.

47. McRee, D.I., Hamrick, P.E. and Zinkl, J. 1975. Some effects of exposure of the Japanese quail embryo to 2450 MHz microwave radiation. Ann. N.Y. Acad. Sci., 247:377.

48. Miller, R.W. 1969. Delayed radiation effects in atomic bomb survivors. Sci., 166:569.

49. Mullenix, P., Norton, S., and Culver, B. 1975. Locomotor damage in rats after x-irradiation in utero. Exp. Neurol., 48:310.

50. Murphree, R., and Pace, H. 1960. The effects of prenatal radiation on postnatal development in rats. Rad. Res., 12;495.

51. Norton, S. 1979. Development of rat telencephalic neurons after prenatal x-irradiation. J. Environ. Hlth. Sci., C13(2):121.

52. Parker, H.M., and Taylor, L.S. 1971. Basic radiation protection criteria. National council on radiation protection and measurement. Report No. 39.

53. Presman, A.S. 1977. Electromagnetic fields and life. Plenum Press, N.Y.C.

54. Rugh, R. 1960. Effects of ionizing radiations on the embryo and/or fetus. In: Errera, M. and Forssberg, A. (eds.), Mechanisms in radiobiology, Academic Press, N.Y.C.

55. Rugh, R. 1973. X-rays and the retina of the primate fetus. Arch. Ophthal., 89:221.

56. Rugh, R. 1976. The relation of sex, age, and weight of mice to microwave radiation sensitivity. J. Microwave Power, 11:127.

57. Rugh, R., Ginns, E.I., Ho, H.S., and Leach, W.M. 1975. Response of the mouse to microwave radiation during estrous cycle and pregnancy. Rad. Res. 62:225.

58. Rugh, R., and Grupp, E. 1960. Fractionated x-irradiation of the mammalian embryo and congenital anomalies. Am. J. Roentgenol., 84:125.

59. Rugh, R., and Wohlfromm, M. 1965. Prenatal x-irradiation and postnatal mortality. Rad. Res., 26:493.

60. Rugh, R., and Wohlfromm, M. 1966. Resistance of the prenatal female mouse to x-ray sterilization. Fertil. Steril., 17:396.

61. Russell, L.B., and Russell, W.L. 1954. An analysis of the changing radiation response of the developing mouse embryo. J. Cell Comp. Physiol., 43(supl. 1):103.

62. Tekeuchi, I., Shoji, R., and Murakami, U. 1976. On the early ultrastructural changes of rat embryonic cerebral mantle after x-irradiation. Annot. Zool. Japon., 49(4):213.

63. Tamaki, Y., and Inouye, M. 1976. Brightness discrimination learning in a skinner box in prenatally x-irradiated rats. Physiol. Behav., 16:343.

64. Tamaki, Y., Shoji, R., Takeuchi, I.K., and Murakami, U. 1976. Facilitatory effect of prenatal x-irradiation on two-way avoidance behavior in rats. Japan. Psychol. Res., 18(3):142.

65. Van Ummerson, C.A. 1963. An experimental study of developmental abnormalities induced in the chick embryo by exposure to radio frequency waves. Ph.D. Dissertation, Department of Biology, Tufts University, Medford, Mass.

66. Vernadakis, A., Curry, J.H., Maletta, G.J., Irvine, G., and Timiras, P.A. 1966. Convulsive responses in prenatally irradiated rats. Exp. Neurol.,16:57.

67. Walker, S., and Furchtgott, E. 1970. Effects of prenatal x-irradiation on the acquisition, extinction, and discrimination of a classically conditioned response. Rad. Res., 42:120.

68. Werboff, J., Broeder, J., Havlena, J., and Sikov, M. 1961. Effects of prenatal x-ray irradiation on audiogenic seizures in the rat. Exp. Neurol., 4:189.

69. Wilson, J.G. 1954. Differentiation and reaction of rat embryos to radiation. J. Cell. Comp. Physiol., 43:11.

70. Wood, J.W., Johnson, K.G., and Omori, Y. 1976. In utero exposure to the hiroshima atomic bomb. An evaluation of head size and mental retardation: twenty years later. Pediat., 39:385.

71. Wood, J.W., Johnson, K.G., Omori, Y., Kawammoto, S., and Keehn, R.J. 1967. Mental retardation in children exposed in utero to the atomic bombs in hiroshima and nagasaki. Am. J. Publ. Hlth., 57:1381.

CHAPTER 7

THE TERATOLOGIST AS A CONSULTANT

By

E. Marshall Johnson, Ph.D.
Professor and Chairman,
Department of Anatomy
Directory, Daniel Baugh Institute
Jefferson Medical College
1020 Locust Street
Philadelphia, Pa. 19107

Consultants are hired for any of a broad range of assignments, although most are in the field of management consulting. There are peculiarities more or less unique to each type of consulting, and I will address only some of the practical aspects and common denominators relevant to consulting in the area of reproductive toxicology and teratology. A Company usually calls upon a consultant for assignments such as review of an experimental protocol, examination of data or advice or opinions regarding a safety evaluation study in experimental animals. This is an area of increasing interest and complexity and it is not uncommon for pharmaceutical and chemical manufacturers to call upon a teratologist to consult on specific problems or questions on such topics. The initial contact is usually made by the in-house teratologist or toxicologist and this is the optimal avenue. When the initial conversation is with middle or upper management, the approach tends to be couched in terms more applicable to a management consultant. On the other hand, when the client's contact person is a scientist, the preliminary discussion more rapidly becomes focused in terms pertinent to the problems. Since consulting presents interesting challenges and educational experiences for both the consultant and the client, it behooves all to get started on the proper foot.

The now familiar questions and situations regarding teratology posed by pharmaceutical manufacturers for many years are beginning to be posed also by the chemical industry. The associated factors or considerations are somewhat different for these two industries but the basic problems and questions are remarkably similar. Expert advice is sought regarding a particular substance, experiment or data base. Frequently the area of concern revolves around a poorly executed or designed study, or ambiguous data and conclusions.

After some eighteen years of occasional consulting as a teratologist, one does develop some perceptions and perhaps these could be shared. I believe that it is by this tenuous thread that I have been asked to briefly address the topic.

WHAT IS PROVIDED BY A CONSULTANT?

Just what does a consultant provide in the realm of safety evaluations for reproduction and teratogenesis? Firstly, one would assume that the person so retained would represent extensive informational and experience background in a very narrow area. There are a great many factors (known and unknown) which impinge on a study involving pregnant animals. The most esoteric appearing nuance may have significant impact upon the interpretation and utilization of experimental data in a study of reproduction and development. The experience that the consultant brings to bear should be specifically oriented toward dealing with these special types of situations and problems. The external consultant may have had repeated experiences with a particular type of problem involving abnormal developmental biology because of the diversity of his consulting contacts. (These experiences might therefore be considerably beyond those of any resident individual whose primary experiences come through the one professional position and its history). The consultant should be expected to give his full attention to the particular problem but only for a limited time and for a well defined task. He/she should act as a resource person hired to solve a particular problem or answer a specific question and then should be willing to step aside and allow the in-house people to use the interpretation as they see fit. This is not to imply that the client should not expect follow-up to be available. It is not uncommon for the such to be sought, sometimes years later.

HOW DOES ONE GO ABOUT
SELECTING A CONSULTANT?

Perhaps the best and most common means of selecting such a resource person is when someone you know and respect can advise you that a particular individual did a good job as a consultant for them. Optimally, several such individuals might be suggested by your various contacts. A prospective consultant can then be contacted either in person or by phone to determine whether or not you can actually work with them. There are many styles for approaching experimental questions or problem areas and you should find an individual who uses a format of operation with which you can be comfortable. Very early in the conversation it is wise to determine whether or not the would-be consultant acutally understands the problem and is comfortable in dealing with such situations. Additionally, it is certainly not untoward to determine whether or not the would-be consultant actually has the skill, experience and *time* to be of help in your particular situation. I think it is very important to stear clear of the 'yes' men in the world. In their effort to be agreeable and to give you the information that they think you might like to have, they may create problems for you which will surface only at some later time. The amount of time a consultant has available is also important and, as the conversation progresses, some definite timeline should begin to evolve. If the prospective consultant does not seem to be *interested in your problem* and does not have a desire to *facilitate your success,* then I think you should move on to the next individual on your list of prospects.

WHAT CAN YOU LOGICALLY EXPECT?

Firstly, you will be working with a very busy person but you should expect his undivided attention for whatever time span you two have agreed upon. Although some teaching and even coaching may be forthcoming, a consultant really is only a person with specialized information and background and the experience to apply it to your particular situation. Miracles are in short supply but you may be favorably surprised how the application of that background or specialized information can significantly alter the problem's magnitude. Many would-be problems are really only poorly executed studies or naively interpreted data.

At an early time, mail the relevant data to the consultant for his confidential study and initial reaction. The more data (within limits) sent to the consultant individual, the more firm can be the ultimate statement. These data should be organized in some logical and readily apparent manner from the statement of the concern, through tabular data statistically analyzed, to the actual unreduced information. The nature of the information sent may vary but some thought should go into its assembly. Some explanation should also accompany the material.

Make optimal use of both the consultant's time and your own time and money. The best way to do this is to keep things moving smoothly and to do your own homework. You can expect a series of questions to be posed to you and you will need to have at your fingertips at least some general grasp of the facts relating to the particular situation. The problem needs to be stated in a clear and honest manner. Focus the consultant's attention as soon as possible. This is usually not a difficult thing to do, as the question probably has been discussed extensively amongst you and your colleagues. Phrase the problem or task in the same general terms used at home. You need to provide a complete set of relevant current data and these should not be intermixed with generalized background or historical information. Some preparation and forethought should be given on your part to the availability of historical summaries because, on the infrequent occasions when they are necessary, these data can be quite valuable. By and large, however, such is not needed. Discuss your own concerns regarding the problem and your aspirations for its resolution either in person or by phone at an early stage of the consultant's involvement.

With logical cooperation regarding the above factors in his/her mind, an experienced consultant can usually give a rather clear and realistic timeline for the number of hours that will be required to review the data and when the initial review will be completed. Initially this will be somewhat tentative, but generally I think you will find that the amount of time required is somewhat less than you may have imagined. After his initial review a consultant should be asked for an interim report, perhaps by phone, to identify problem areas and to make sure that he/she is properly focused on your areas of concern. At the same time the consultant should be able to discuss with you any related topics or considerations that may have come out of this study. I personally do not feel that it is wise to have a consultant submit the final report in writing at this time. It is much better to have a rough draft submitted so you and your colleagues can review it at leisure. The consultant can be contacted by phone or in writing prior to preparing a final report. This is not to imply that the facts or their basic meaning will be changed. There may be, however, considerations or related data that can affect the certainty or confidence level which could be discussed further at the time of the preliminary draft. It is very important that you feel free to discuss and explain items of particular interest at any stage during the review process. You must not fall into the trap of expecting an extramural consultant to be intimately familiar with your shop. Explain the in-house situation but only to the extent you feel it will benefit the scientific resolution of the problem. Before I leave this topic, a few last suggestions. 1) Make sure you yourself are available so that the consultant will be able to query you on a specific point expeditiously. 2) Have a single primary contact person. This is highly recommended or conflicting signals will go to the consultant and dilute the direction of his attention. 3) After you receive the final report, if you feel that you do not fully understand some of the bases on which the document is written, feel free to recontact the consultant.

Afterwards, I think you should do a postmortum. Some of the questions you would want to ask yourself at this point would be what happened, what did not happen, and how did this affect the final outcome. Consider whether or not you brought in the correct consultant and whether it was done at the proper time. Determine if the problem was stated clearly and whether you provided the data in a timely manner. On the other side of the coin, you should consider whether or not the consultant efficiently and effectively grasped and understood the situation and whether or not the task was approached in a professional manner. Did the report arrive on time and did it clearly address the central issue which was the reason for your contacting him in the first place. Last, but not least, I think you will want to ask yourself if you and your firm benefitted from the effort.

CHAPTER 8

ASSESSMENT OF REPRODUCTIVITY TOXICITY - "STATE OF THE ART"

Mildred S. Christian, Ph.D.
Argus Research Laboratories, Inc.
2025 Ridge Road
Perkasie, Pennsylvania 18944

INTRODUCTION

Reproductive toxicity assessment has become relatively standardized. The procedures proposed by the United States Environmental Protection Agency (EPA) (1,2), Japan (3), Great Britain (4), the Organization for Economic Cooperation and Development (OECD) an international organization of 23 countries (5) and the United States Interagency Regulatory Liaison Group (IRLG) an organization of six Federal agencies (6) are all essentially based on the 1966 Food and Drug Agency (FDA) Guidelines (7). These have been frequently and well described (8, 9) and are essentially designed to encompass the critical periods for reproductive hazard (10). Minor variations exist in the procedures proposed by the various regulatory agencies, in the number of tests required and in the interpretation of these regulations.

A summary of the various required assessments is given in Table 1. The table was developed on the basis of statements in the various guidelines and other sources (11).

Because the 1966 FDA procedures have been permitted to remain guidelines, rather than directives, it is still possible to interpret and vary procedures, while performing an adequate, or even improved study. The following is a brief outline of my interpretation of the procedures for performing the FDA series of tests.

The FDA approach to reproductive hazard assessment has been to perform a three segment evaluation. These reproductive studies are commonly referred to as Segments I, II and III.

TABLE 1

	SEGMENT I	SEGMENT II	SEGMENT III	REPRODUCTION (2 or 3 GENERATIONS)
FDA (1966)	M,F 1 SPECIES	F - 1 RODENT (20) F - 1 NON-RODENT (10)	F - 1 RODENT	F - 1 RODENT
EPA (PROPOSED FIFRA; 1978 TSCA; 1979)	--	F - 2 SPECIES (RODENT -20; NON-RODENT - 12)	--	--
JAPAN (1975	M, F 1 SPECIES	F - 1 RODENT (30) BEHAVIOR	F - 1 RODENT BEHAVIOR	F - 1 RODENT BEHAVIOR
GREAT BRITAIN (1974)	M, F 1 SPECIES SKELETAL, VISCERAL AND BEHAVIORAL	F - 1 RODENT (24) F - 1 NON-RODENT (12) MAY NOW WANT BEHAVIOR	F - 1 RODENT	F - RODENT BEHAVIOR "POSSIBLE"
OECD (1979)	--	F - 1 RODENT (20) F - 1 NON-RODENT (12)	--	--
IRLG (1981)	--	F - 1 RODENT (20) F - 1 NON-RODENT (15)	--	--

M = MALE; F = FEMALE ( ) = NUMBER OF ANIMALS TO BE EVALUATED

DESCRIPTION OF PROTOCOLS

Segment I Evaluations

FDA

The Segment I study evaluates effects on fertility and general reproductive performance. It is used to assess toxic effects of the test agent on gonadal function and mating behavior in both male and female test animals as well as conception rates, the early and late stages of gestation, parturition, lactation and finally, development of offspring. The results of this study generally are used for planning the Segment II and III evaluations in the same species.

The Segment I study is the only evaluation of reproductive toxicity performed in the male. An important point frequently missed is that the male animal is the unit tested. A minimum of 20 male and 20 female rodents, usually rats, should be assigned to a control and each of three agent-treated dosage groups. To determine whether there is a sex difference in reproductive toxicity or a potentiation of effect when both sexes are administered the test agent, it has been suggested (12) that an additional group of ten male and ten female rats be assigned to both the control and high dosage groups.

All rats should be sexually mature when assigned to study. Male rats should be administered the test agent for a minimum of 60 days prior to and then through a cohabitation period. Female rats should be evaluated for regular estrous cycling by daily examination of smears of vaginal contents, prior to initiation of treatment. These female rats should then be administered the test agent for 14 days prior to cohabitation and estrous cycling similarly evaluated during this period. Treatment of female rats should continue until the rats are sacrificed and Caesarean-sectioned on day 13 of presumed gestation, after observation of non-pregnancy (greater than 25 days of presumed gestation) or after natural delivery and weaning of pups. The supplemental control and high dosage group rats should be placed in cohabitation with each other, and all of these female rats permitted to naturally deliver and nurse pups.

One male and one female rat should be used in initial matings. Mating performance of male and female rats should be evaluated on the basis of observation of either spermatozoa in a daily smear of vaginal contents and/or a copulation plug. Day 0 of gestation should be defined as the day on which insemination is confirmed.

One-half of the female rats in each dosage group, selected randomly or on an odd-even basis, should be sacrificed on day 13 of presumed gestation and examined for number and distribution of corpora lutea, implantations and live and resorbing embryos. Any condition in either the dam or sire which may have contributed to reduced fertility should be noted.

The remaining one-half of the female rats in each dosage group should be permitted to naturally deliver and nurse offspring. The duration of gestation should be evaluated. Litters should be examined for number, viability, gender, body weight and gross morphological variations in pups. Maternal and pup survival and body weight should be recorded at birth and on days 4, 7, 14 and 21 postparturition (birth = day 1). To standardize litters, random culling, preferably to four male and four female pups per litter, may be done on day 4 postparturition. Stillborn or moribund pups may be preserved for additional studies.

VARIATIONS

Japan

The protocol to be followed for submission to Japanese regulatory agencies is essentially the same as that proposed by the FDA except that maternal treatment is stopped at the stage of initiation of major organogenesis. This treatment is stopped in the rat on day 6 and in the mouse on day 7 of gestation.

Great Britain

British regulatory agencies require a slight alteration of the FDA protocol. Rather than terminating one-half of the dams on day 13 of presumed gestation, these rats are Caesarean-sectioned on day 20 of presumed gestaton. Fetuses are examined not only for viability, as in the day 13 evaluation, but also for gross external defects. The fetuses are preserved for possible examination for soft tissue and skeletal variations. Naturally delivered litters are not terminated at weaning; selected pups are continued on study beyond 21 days postparturition and then evaluated for general sensory (auditory, visual) and "behavioral" development and fertility.

EPA, OECD and IRLG

These regulatory agencies do not currently require Segment I evaluations.

SEGMENT II EVALUATIONS

FDA

Segment II studies are designed to evaluate the teratogenic potential of a test agent. FDA segment II evaluations are performed, in both a rodent and a non-rodent species, most frequently the rat and rabbit. Males used for breeding are not administered the test agent. Standardly, day 0 of presumed gestation is the day spermatozoa, a vaginal plug (rats, mice) or insemination (rabbits) occurs. Animals are treated during the period of major organogenesis and Caesarean-sectioned one or two days prior to the expected time of natural delivery. Treatment periods for commonly used species are:

Test Species	Treatment Period (Days of Gestation)	C-Sectioned (Day)
RODENT		
Rat	6 - 15	20
Mouse	6 - 15	18
Hamster	6 - 12	15

Test Species	Treatment Period (Days of Gestation)	C-Sectioned (Day)
NON-RODENT		
Rabbit	6 - 18	29 or 30

Following maternal Caesarean-sectioning, the uterus is examined for number and placement of implantations, early and late resorptions, and live and dead fetuses. Ovaries are examined for the number of corpora lutea.

All fetuses are weighed and examined for gross external variations and gender. In rodent studies, one-third of the fetuses in each litter are assigned to soft tissue examination using standardly accepted methods such as Wilson's sectioning technique (13) or Staples' visceral examination technique (14). The remaining two-third's of the fetuses in each litter are examined for skeletal variations after staining with alizarin red-S (15).

In non-rodent studies, all fetuses are examined for soft-tissue and skeletal malformations.

The FDA suggest 20 rodents and 10 non-rodents per dosage group and a control and three dosage levels in rodent studies, with only a control and two dosage levels in non-rodent studies.

VARIATIONS

Recommended Practices

When these treatment periods were originally suggested in 1966, the time of implantation in the various species was not accurately known. Initiation of treatment after histologic implantation has occurred, rather than simply nidation, ensures that the compound is being tested for its teratogenic potential and not for its ability to interfere with implantation. If the landmarks used for the period of major organogenesis are from histologic implantation to palatal closure (16), the appropriate treatment time for use in a study of teratogenic potential, the exposure periods for the various species should be as follows:

Test Species	Treatment Period (Days of Gestation)
RODENT	
Rat	7 - 15
Mouse	7 - 15
Hamster	6 - 12
NON—RODENT	
Rabbit	8 - 19

Although not stated as required in the guidelines, it seems appropriate that the minimum number of female animals cited for evaluation, for example, 20 per dosage group, should be pregnant. It is obviously not possible to evaluate teratogenic potential of a test agent in non-pregnant animals.

Another recommendation is to standardly evaluate three, rather than two, dosage levels of the test agent in non-rodents, in order to better determine a dosage response. This approach has been adopted by all other regulatory bodies.

EPA

The EPA protocols differ from those of the FDA in that two species, not necessarily rodent and non-rodent, are required. In EPA studies, one-half of the fetuses in each litter are assigned to soft tissue evaluations, and the other one-half of these fetuses to skeletal evaluation. Minor additional evaluations such as placental, uterine and maternal carcass weights are suggested, although the variability of these parameters makes them inappropriate for evaluation.

The most significant difference between the protocols proposed for Segment II evaluations by the EPA, and those suggested by the FDA, is that in the EPA protocols the treatment period is extended to the day prior to maternal Caesarean-sectioning. This change was made on the hypothesis that treatment during both the embryonal and fetal periods will increase the probability of demonstrating an agent's teratogenic potential. Thus, the EPA protocols have the following treatment time requirements:

Test Species	Treatment Period (Days of Gestation)	C-Sectioned (Day)
Rat	6 - 19	20
Mouse	6 - 17	18
Hamster	6 - 14	15
Rabbit	6 - 28 or 29	29 or 30

This procedure does not seem appropriate for the following reasons:

1. Prolonged treatment may result in enzyme induction or suppression, and thereby alter effects of the test agent;

2. Prolonged treatment may result in increased maternal toxic response and thus require that lower maximal dosages be evaluated;

3. Extending the treatment period into the time of fetal growth, beyond the period when major embryogenesis occurs, will most probably result in functional changes which would not be detected in gross morphological evaluations. The literature indicates that functional, rather than gross morphological, changes are associated with fetal insult (17). These changes may be detected in functional evaluations performed postnatally, but they would not be apparent in fetuses evaluated at term for altered organogenesis or ossification.

4. There is a high probability that the number of fetal deaths will be in-

creased by prolonging treatment, with a resultant loss of fetal material available for examination.

5. Prolonging the treatment time increases the cost of performing the study without a significant gain in information.

Japan

The Japanese require that 30 rodents be evaluated per dosage group. Rats are treated days 7 through 17 of gestation. Twenty dams are Caesarean-sectioned on day 20 of gestation, and 10 dams are permitted to naturally deliver litters. Postnatal evaluation of maturation and physical development is required as well as some measurement of locomotion, learning, sensory function or emotionality. Fertility on the F1 generation is evaluated as well as the gross anatomical developmental state of F2 generation fetuses.

Great Britain

The British recommend 24 rodents and 12 non-rodents per dosage group, although the requirement may be increased to 20 non-rodents per dosage group. In certain cases (undefined), postnatal "behavioral" evaluations are required.

OECD

These guidelines currently recommend 20 pregnant rodent and 12 pregnant non-rodent animals in each dosage group.

IRLG

At present, the IRLG guidelines require 20 pregnant rodent and 15 pregnant non-rodent animals in each dosage group.

SEGMENT III EVALUATIONS

FDA

The peri- and post-natal evaluation is designed to evaluate the effects of a test agent on the development of the fetus during the last one-third of gestation and any adverse effects on delivery, lactation and postparturition pup development. The study is usually performed in rats. Dams are mated by male breeders which are not exposed to the test agent. The dams are treated with the test agent beginning on day 15 of presumed gestation and continuing through delivery and 21 days postparturition. The duration of gestation, delivery, any complications observed at parturition and the number and viability of naturally delivered litters are evaluated. If poor pup survival occurred in the Segment I evaluation of the test agent, cross-fostering of a group of control and high dosage group litters is frequently added.

Japan

For submission to Japanese regulation agencies, the FDA designed protocol is prolonged to include "behavioral" evaluations of F1 generation pups, in order to examine postnatal development.

EPA, IRLG, and OECD

The Segment III evaluation is not currently required by these regulatory groups.

REPRODUCTION (2 OR 3 GENERATIONS) EVALUATIONS

FDA and EPA

The studies are generally performed when food additives are evaluated (FDA) or as the third study for submission of agents regulated by the EPA. The EPA generally uses this test as the replacement for the FDA Segment I and Segment III evaluations.

The F0 generation consists of young rodents in which treatment is initiated immediately following weaning and continues through mating, delivery and nursing of the F1 generation pups. A second mating of the F0 parental generation may be evaluated. The F1 generation pups are individually treated after weaning, which usually occurs at 21 days of age. Treatment of these rats continues through mating and delivery of F2 generation pups.

Primary differences between the FDA and EPA protocols are whether two (EPA) or three (FDA) generations are evaluated and the extent of histopathology requirements. The FDA protocol requires target organ evaluation, while the EPA protocol requires histopathology of all organ systems.

Japan and Great Britain

The Japanese require postnatal "behavioral" assessment, and the British have "behavior" as a possible additional requirement. Submission of food and water consumption data, ophthalmologic evaluations and organ weight data are frequently requested.

IRLG and OECD

Reproduction evaluation guidelines are not yet used by these groups.

DISCUSSION OF PROTOCOLS
WITH RECOMMENDATIONS

The major variations among the protocols designed by the various regulatory bodies have been addressed in the previous section. The following is an overview of some of the problems observed by myself and others (18), and some suggestions for future risk assessment.

The greatest number of compounds which have not been evaluated for reproductive hazard also have not been evaluated for other toxic risks. Chemical manufacturers presently bear the greatest burden for determining hazards. These manufacturers generally are required to perform studies using the EPA Proposed Guidelines (FIFRA or TSCA). Due to the current economic and regulatory climate, the number of agents to be evaluated and the number of tests to be performed far exceed the number of rats and scientists available to perform these evaluations. As a result, for regulatory purposes, a political/economic, not a scientific, decision must be made to determine the greatest hazard.

The socio-political climate in which testing must be performed has changed because the public is now aware of some of the problems associated with exposure to toxic agents. Actually, the public was always aware that problems existed, but the current climate is different because the public is now demanding protection. Because of this clamor for protection, there are at least three government committees developing risk assessment programs which primarily emphasize environmental reproductive hazards. Two are in the EPA and one in the IRLG. The Equal Employment Opportunity Commission (EEOC) is proposing that balanced research on reproductive hazard be performed on existing substances in the workplace, as well as on new products. The FDA is proposing that toxic effects of a drug on male fertility be evaluated, in addition to performing subacute studies, before phase I clinical trials are initiated.

An additional economic factor is that the public also wants new products. Many of the regulations imposed on development of new products require a "no effect" level. The manufacturing community is in the untenable position of either using screens which show "no effect", or using more sensitive screens with the possible end result of prohibition from further development of the product.

Scientifically, our tests must be clarified. Our currently practiced evaluations confuse endpoints, and regulation must be based on the endpoint. A prime example of a confounding evaluation is the TSCA and FIFRA EPA two generation evaluation of reproduction. As currently proposed, it is not a good test of reproduction. It also is not a good test of carcinogenic potential. Like Topsy, it simply grew. The procedure developed from the old format used for nutritional studies, in which it was considered appropriate to use several generations of animals to evaluate the effects of prolonged undernutrition. The endpoint was reduced litter size. In 1970, the FDA proposed that the accumulation of toxins could be appropriately evaluated in this paradime, because accumulation of toxins was considered to be the reverse of loss of nutrients (19). The EPA protocols have added extensive necropsy and histopathology procedures, making the study really a short-term chronic toxicity/carcinogenicity evaluation. This significant increase in evaluation requirements was proposed by the EPA even though long-term carcinogenicity evaluations in two species, the in-life portions of which each require 18 months to two years to perform, were already part of the submission package.

Extension of the Segment II teratology evaluation, as proposed by FIFRA and TSCA, to include treatment during both embryonal and fetal growth, and the collection of additional Caesarean-sectioning measurements only confound interpretation of the data. Abortions will be increased in all study groups, metabolic changes may be produced, lower dosages may be required for use and data which cannot be interpreted will be collected.

Each of the currently used screens have major obvious design deficiences, some of which were discussed. In general, new protocol designs have incorporated the old defects. In addition, new measurements, such as "behavioral" evaluations (20, 21) have been added to the old screens. These new observations may obscure even those few endpoints which could be validated: life, death and gross anatomical malformation.

The important facts to be recognized are:

(1) We must accept that regulation and risk assessment will of necessity have to be based not on the most subtle effect of an agent, but rather on the most toxic effect.

(2) We must stop adding onto existing methodology and making even the end points which we can validate obscure.

(3) We must also accept that current economic/social pressure requires rapid validation and use of screening techniques which answer single, or at most several, questions.

The necessary standardization and validation of end points which are more subtle than life and death are currently unavailable. We are performing evaluations in species which are different from man. We are using long-term evaluations which provide valid, reproducible information in test species only at the levels of life, death and gross change. Thus, it is not possible to extrapolate the animal test results to man.

No one would disagree with the concept that an inexpensive test, or a series of tests, which are valid and which could be extrapolated to man. There does not appear to be any way in which the huge burden of research required can be accomplished using current techniques.

The first step in resolving this dilemma is to alter the concept of risk assessment. To change this concept, re-education of the scientific and regulatory communities is required, prior to re-education of the general public.

Risk assessment of agents must be based on regulation of an agent according to its most toxic effect. If an agent is a carcinogen, it should be regulated on the basis of this hazard. If it is a non-carcinogen, and its specific hazard is teratogenicity, it should be regulated on its teratogenic potential. The volume of work can only be approached through initial classification on the basis of the most significant hazard. Only by developing more appropriate screening techniques, can the possibility of completing the task exist.

REFERENCES

1. Environmental Protection Agency.: Pesticide Programs, Proposed Guidelines for Registering Pesticides in the U.S.; Hazard Evaluation: Humans and Domestic Animals Federal Register, Part II, 43(163):163.83-3 Teratogenicity studies; 163.83-4 Reproduction study, Tuesday, August 22, 1978.
2. Environmental Protection Agency.: Proposed Health Effects Test Standards for Toxic Substances Control Act Test Rules and Proposed Good Laboratory Practice Standards for Health Effects. Federal Register, Part IV, 44(145): Subpart F-Teratogenic/Reproductive Health Effects: 772.116-1 General; 772.116-2 Teratogenic effects test standards; 772.116-3 Reproductive effects test standards, Thursday, July 26, 1979.
3. Yakushin No. 529.: On animal experimental methods for testing the effects of drugs on reproduction. Head of Evaluation and Registration Division and Head of Biological Pharmaceutical Preparation Division, Pharmaceutical and Supply Bureau, Ministry of Health and Welfare, Japan, 1975.
4. Committee on the Safety of Medicines.: Notes for guidance on reproduction studies. Department of Health and Social Security, Great Britain, 1974.
5. Organization for Economic Cooperation and Development (OECD).: Final Report - OECD Short Term and Long Term Toxicology Groups, Teratogenicity, 110-113, December 31, 1979.
6. Interagency Regulatory Liaison Group (IRLG).: Recommended Guideline for Teratogenicity Studies in the Rat, Mouse, Hamster or Rabbit, April, 1980.
7. Food and Drug Administration.: Guidelines for Reproductive Studies for Safety Evaluation of Drugs for Human Use. Washington, D.C., 1966.
8. Palmer, A.K.; Some thoughts on reproductive studies for safety evaluations. Proc. Euro. Soc. Study Drug Tox. 14:79-90, 1973.
9. Tuchmann-Duplessis, H.: Teratogenic drug screening. Present procedures and requirements. Teratology 5:271-286, 1972.
10. Goldman, A.S.: Critical periods of prenatal toxicity. Clinical in Perinatology 6(2):203-218, 1979.
11. Sher, S.P., Bokelman, D.L. and Ditzler, W.D.: Preclinical toxicity requirements for human drugs. Drug Inf. J. 14(2):82-97, 1980.
12. Staples, R.E.: personal communication, 1980.

13. Wilson, J.G.: Methods for administering agents and detecting malformations in experimental animals. *Teratology, Principles and Techniques* Wilson, J.G. and Warkany, J. (eds.), Un. Chicago Press, Chicago, pp. 262-277, 1965.

14. Staples, R.E.: detection of visceral alterations in mammalian fetuses. Teratology 9(3):37A-38A, 1974.

15. Staples, R.E. and Schnell, J.L.: Refinement in rapid clearing technic in the KOH-alizarin red S method for fetal bone. Stain Technol. 39:61-63, 1963.

16. Shepard, T.H.: *Catolog of Teratogenic Agents.* John Hopkins University Press, Baltimore, MD. 410 pp.

17. Christian, M.S.: Postnatal alteration of gastrointestinal physiology, hematology, clinical chemistry and other non-CNS parameters. In: *Handbook of Experimental Pharmacology; Teratogenesis and Reproductive Toxicology,* Johnson, E.M. and Kochar, D.M. (eds.), Springer-Verlag, in press.

18. Schwetz, B.A. and Rao, K.S.: Insensitivity of tests for reproductive problems. J. Environ. Path. Toxicol. 3:81-98, 1980.

19. Food and Drug Administration Advisory Committee on Protocols for Safety Evaluations; Panel on Reproduction.: Report on reproduction studies in the safety evaluation of food additives and pesticide residues. Toxicol. Appl. Pharmacol. 16:264-296, 1970.

20. Buelke-Sam, J. and Kimmel, C.A.: Development and standardization of screening methods for behavioral teratology. Teratology 20:17-30, 1979.

21. Coyle, I., Wayner, M.J., and Singer, G.: Theoretical Review. Behavioral teratogenesis: A critical evaluation. Pharmacol. Biochem. Behav. 4(2): 191-200, 1976.

CHAPTER 9

PRACTICAL APPLICATION OF SYSTEMS FOR RAPID DETECTION OF POTENTIAL TERATOGENIC HAZARDS

E. Marshall Johnson, Ph.D.
Daniel Baugh Institute
Jefferson Medical College
1020 Locust Street
Philadelphia, PA 19107

There are as many as 60,000 chemical substances in our environment at the present time and each year at least 300 new materials are added to the milieu in which we live. There is an equally large or perhaps larger group of substances which are restricted to research laboratories or exist only within the pipes and reaction vessels of chemical manufacturers. These chemicals are esoteric items of interest to researchers or are intermediates of step-wise procedures in the chemical industry. Neither class would be considered as posing a hazard because of their small quantity and lack of dissemination.

Only several hundred (15) substances have been investigated to even a minor extent regarding the degree to which they potentially *could* pose a hazard to the conceptus. We are essentially or even totally ignorant of any potential hazards which may or may not be posed by any of the remainder. If all the world's developmental toxicologists were employed full-time, it might be possible to examine up to 200 substances per year. Obviously new materials would still be introduced at a more rapid rate than they could be examined and, furthermore, the cost would be too great in both money and allocation of resources. All of the foregoing assumes that testing for adverse affects on the conceptus will continue to be only by the screening methods currently available (14). These studies have been in general use since the mid- or late 1960's and each requires large numbers of pregnant animals and considerable effort from skilled technical personnel.

Development of reliable and rapid prescreening systems would overcome the rather dark scenarit just alluded to and, in addition, would have benefits perhaps less obvious on first glance. The principal advantage of a prescreening system for teratogenic hazards would be to protect the unborn human from maldevelopment. That is, a prescreen would permit examination of large numbers of the existing substances in a relatively short time and allow detection of those which actually are hazardous to developmental events.Most substances do not pose significant hazards to the conceptus because they are really no more toxic to development of an embryo than they are to the adult organism and so exposure is permitted at doses below the adult toxic level. It is important to remember that every substance has the potential to disrupt development of the conceptus (8) but most agents exhibit this ability only at doses also toxic to the adult. They are coeffective teratogens (7) and once this is established they need not be examined further for their teratogenic ability except where specific needs exist, e.g. substances to be used primarily by women of childbearing age. One of the primary advantages of a prescreening system would be to prioritize substances into groups deserving further study regarding teratology while permitting the majority to continue in our environment regulated only on the basis of adult toxicity. This is acceptable once it has been established that they pose no unique threat to developmental events. This latter assumes, of course, that such agents will be examined for other toxic effects and exposure will be controlled on the basis of toxicity to the adult. For such compounds application of a safety factor would provide, of itself, protection for the conceptus at least equal to that protection being offered to the adult because the substances are coeffective teratogens lacking significant hazard potential (5). If we do not acquire a prescreen for potential developmental hazards, we cannot provide the same degree of safety to the conceptus that is provided the adult. Furthermore, with the current state of affairs the protection which we offer to the conceptus is going to lag increasingly behind that being provided for ourselves - the adults.

A rapid screening system or series of tests for teratogenic potential also would have significant advantages in the world of commerce. When faced with a series of molecules or substitution forms, any one or few of which could serve a particular commercial goal, the industrial toxicologists cannot adequately advise management which of these substances to develop and which to place on the shelf because they are potential teratogenic hazards. Such delineations of potential cannot be predicted by simple inspection of the molecule but a rapid prescreen would allow the industrial toxicologists a scientific basis on which to predict that a particular substance will or will not pose a hazard to the conceptus if it should be released into the environment at some later time. With such information in hand the commercial enterprise can then proceed with some degree of confidence that the compound will not be precluded from use at a later date by an experiment in rodents showing that it is a potential teratogenic hazard.

A related aspect should not be overlooked either and this is that the extent to which two or more substances may or may not interact in some additive or synergistic way to disrupt the conceptus usually cannot be predicted without live animal testing. Such possibilities are real, though seldom discussed, and it could be that it is in this realm of interactions that the human conceptus is presently being placed at the most significant risk.

Last, but not least, the field of teratology would similarly benefit by development of prescreening systems. Any group of prescreens will probably span a significant portion of basic normal and abnormal developmental biology. It follows then that a rapid screening system to examine abnormal developmental sequences will facilitate our study of mechanisms of teratogenesis by making them more readily available for closer examination. Understanding mechanisms permits our examining the effects of agents on specific and essential developmental events and this is the level of understanding prerequisite to successfully avoid being mislead by effects in animals and man which appear superficially similar but really lack etiological relationship.

In the past few years there has been marked interest and effort placed in developing applicable prescreening methods. Some of these are explorations of methods and systems studied in some considerable detail during the 50's and 60's and are novel for uses for old systems. The number of newer concepts and ideas also is growing and some proportioning of these two approaches may have real use for prescreening. Detailed explanations of each of the many systems being advanced with greater or lesser enthusiasm will not be provided here. Attention will be directed to explain those systems which are already available and seem to have some degree of utility. Though each of the systems discussed needs more study and examination for validity, each has already demonstrated some ability for practical application. Two of these systems are *in vivo* methods, one in an *in vitro* system, and two are combinations of each approach. The five systems to be considered are listed in Table 1 along with some of their possible abilities.

In the simplified or abbreviated Segment II (3) procedure the test compound is administered to timed pregnant mice from day 8-12 of gestation and the dams' weight gains during pregnancy are recorded. After natural delivery, the pups are counted and weighed on days 1 and 3. If delivery does not occur the dams are autopsied on this estimated postnatal day 3 and the uterine contents examined for resorption sites. Dose selection by these investigators was determined by either of two methods with the goal of administering the test substance at one dose level, which was wisely chosen to be at or near that producing overt maternal toxicity. The first method for selection of the single dose level to be tested was applied to substances of known teratogenic potential, in which case the level was gleaned from the published literature. The second method for dose selection was applied to substances on which there was no published literature dealing with the teratogenic potential of the substance in question. This dose was selected on the basis of a preliminary range-finding study in adult animals to determine the dose producing the desired degree of overt toxicity in the adult.

This system of Chernof and Kavloch has several rather obvious advantages. It employs familiar animals with methods familiar to all and an impressive number of chemicals has been evaluated by this method. As any other system, it has also some obvious disadvantages and inherent weaknesses. These may be more obvious here because this is a test with a long, though largely unpublished history. It is the type of experiment per-

TABLE I

SYSTEMS	NATURE OF EVALUATION	POTENTIAL DETECTING ABILITIES	REFERENCE
Simplified Segment II (Chernof)	in vivo	Determination of adult and embryo - toxic dose levels	Chernof & Kavlock '80
Serum & Embryos	in vivo + in vitro	Identify Specific Individual Risks	Chatot et al. '80
Homeotic Shifts	in vivo	Predict Adverse Effects in Susceptible Populations and Determine effects due to Low-level Exposure	Russel '79
Organ Culture	in vivo + in vitro	Compare the embryo Toxicity Levels of two or more Substances	Kochhar '75
Hydra attenuata	in vitro	Prediction of Hazard Potential	Johnson '80b

formed by an experimental teratologist to insure that an agent coming under study is actually capable of disrupting *in utero* development at some usable dose level. The system should not be overly criticized just because it is one more familiar to most teratologists. In spite of real or imagined drawbacks the system is somewhat comparable to the more standard and detailed tests in its ability to detect some proportion of the potential teratogenic hazards. When definitive publications appear, there will be a better opportunity to evaluate the actual data but some degree of applicability is to be expected.

Norman Klein and co-investigators (2) have reported that serum of women exposed to teratogens will not adequately support the *in vitro* development of rat embryos. Head-fold-stage rat embryos were collected and cultured on serum derived from persons receiving chemotherapy or anticonvulsants. Timed-pregnant rats were killed at 9.5 days gestation and their intact embryos, along with the associated yolk sacs and ectoplacental cones, were cultured with gluccse-supplemented human serum for 48 hours. There was an increased evidence of death and developmental disturbance among embryos cultured on sera from persons receiving either of the clinical treatments; additionally altered were protein and DNA content per embryo.

Some false positives and potential false negatives may have been identified by the system but the possible errors (if they were errors) of detection were largely on the conservative side. That is, an indication of toxicity where no exposure was known. This is possibly the most intriguing of the possible systems and, though it is not really a prescreen, it has possibilities too great to overlook. When more fully explored, it may actually be able to detect individual persons in individual environments who are at risk. There is, in my view, at least the possibility that it could detect the person at greatest risk in such situations and such valuable possibilities merit close examination.

The third system is also somewhat familiar because it employs live rodents but it represents some very sophisticated thinking by an accomplished developmental biologist. This is the application of the concept of homeosis as a prescreening system described by Dr. Liane B. Russel (13). Homeotic shifts are an old and interesting concept of developmental biology not widely understood or even known, namely that developing organs or organ fields have developmental potencies not normally expressed (16). This was applied by Dr. Russel to animals having marked tendencies toward instability in the developmental potencies expressed by various embryonic anlagen. The concept of homeostatis is best explained by the familiar example of development of mouth parts vis-a-vis limbs by various segments of the insect body. Even though these segments have the full developmental potential to also develop into limbs, they instead express the genome sequences for mouth part formation. Dr. Russel uses the same concept but in the BALB/c mouse which has a marked propensity for instability in the development of several structures (12). One such instability is location of the thoraco-lumbar border. Addition of low levels of a rather weak teratogen shifts this border caudally and the result is manifest as a 14th pair of (lumbar) ribs being expressed in a significant number of the treated litters. These are visualized and identified on clearing and staining by alizarin.

There is a major advantage to this very clever system because the teratogenic potential of a test substance can be quantified objectively to the amount of gama radiation necessary to produce an equivalent homeotic shift (13) in the same strain of animals. This is a significant factor and may more than outweigh the fact that the system perhaps is somewhat labor intensive.

Organ culture has not been extensively studied but it too has several potential advantages for prescreening and should be discussed if my goal is to highlight prescreens which I feel have some demonstrated potential. Methods for limb bud cultures have been described adequately (9) and the potential of limb buds should be considered carefully in comparisons to culture of whole embryos (11).

Timed-pregnant animals (mice in this laboratory) are killed on day 11 of gestation and the embryonic limb buds dissected free of the body just lateral to the somites. The limbs are introduced into a culture chamber on a portion of 25 um thick Millipore filter which is in turn suspended on an appropriate culture medium. The limb buds grow for a maximum of 9 days in culture at which time cartilage models of the bones and some muscle fibers are evident. Development *in vitro* was not fully equivalent to that *in vivo* but treatment with a teratogen elicited similar responses regardless of whether development continued *in vivo* or *in vitro*. An interesting advantage to the *in vitro* limb bud system proposed by Dr. Kochhar is that maternal metabolism of the drug is precluded, thereby permitting direct assessment of the active forms' effects. The limb bud system itself may also have a few drawbacks but within limits there may be applications for determining the relative potency of two or more substances for disrupting those developmental events occuring in limb buds.

The applicability of whole embryo culture to teratogenic screening, I think, is limited from wide application from the view point of its being very labor intensive and the fact that the embryo does not develop normally for any extended period even at the anatomical level. The basic problem probably has to do with cellular respiration and availability of nutrients.

An additional prescreening system is that employing the fresh water coelenterate *Hydra attenuata*. This organism is uniquely situated in the animal kingdom in that it is the most primitive form composed of complex tissues and organs yet it is the highest animal form capable of total whole body regeneration. When adult *Hydra attenuata* are disassociated into their component cells, these cells can be randomly reaggregated (4) into an artificial "embryo" (6) which under normal circumstances will regenerate new adult animals within about a week. During this process of total whole body regeneration this artificial embryo must achieve most, if not all, of the developmental phenomenon required during real embryogenesis. This system is depicted in figures 1 and 2 which indicate some of the more easily recognizable developmental phenomena which occur in this artificial embryo.

The interesting aspect is that various chemicals adversely affect one or more of these developmental events and result in abnormal development recognizable on simple inspection of fresh specimens at low magnification. The dose or concentration of test material needed to achieve this abnormal development may bear no direct relationship to that needed to disrupt the developmental events in mammals. However, this lowest developmental-disruptive dose can be the denominator of a ratio of some use; the numerator being the dose or concentration toxic to the intact adult *Hydra attenuata*. Typical data and the calculated ratios by this system are listed in Table 2.

To determine the degree of validity (or lack thereof) for these data it is necessary to compare them with that developed by studies in rodents. Such data are arranged in Table 3 where the lowest teratogenic and adult toxic doses available from mammals is similarly calculated as the A/D ratio. When the two lists are compared with one another, the hydra system has apparently done an interesting job of correctly ranking the substances into generally the same type of increasing teratogenic hazard sequences as did the rodents. There are two main differences: first, hydra tends to over estimate the degree of hazard as one moves to the increasingly potent teratogens, and second the cost in time and resources of developing the data in hydra is about 1/10 of the cost of the data developed in rodents. This system appears especially amenable to determing which of a larger list of substances are going to pose teratogenic hazards and which will not. This would seem of particular interest to chemical manufacturers because, not only can it be determined whether or not a particular substance is a developmental hazard, but they can also choose the most promising compound for development from among a group of substances which are all acceptable for a particular application.

Neither individually nor collectively do the systems described come even close to meeting the various sets of characteristics some have listed for a teratology prescreen. Such lists were perhaps of some use in stimulating thought or providing direction at one time, but actually they are quite irrelevant. A rose bush meets none of the various criteria such as having a placenta, etc., yet it might become a useable screen. If a test substance were poured onto a rose bush, the bush would respond in some manner. A dose response relationship could even be developed between the concentration of test substance and the bushes' response. This would be an absolutely acceptable prescreen of teratogenic potential regardless of factors such as absorption and excretion if the system could meet one condition. It would have to predict what the effects of the compound were when it was administered to mammals in the more standard screening systems. Therein lies the problem. One cannot be optimistic regarding the possibilities of predicting accurate-

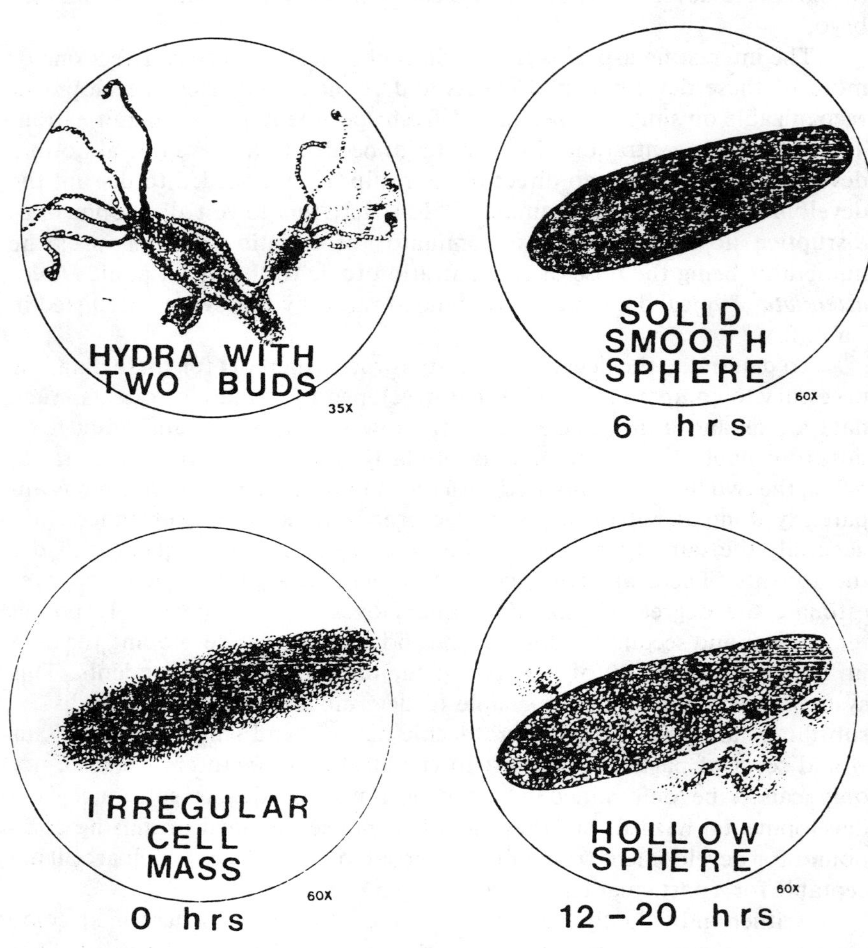

FIGURE 1   Diagrammatic representation of adult **Hydra attenuata** and the beginning of total whole body regeneration.

Upper Left - An adult polyp reproducing asexually by means of lateral buds.

Lower Left - The dissociated cells of several adult **Hydra attenuata** are packed by gentle centrifugation and at 0 hours are randomly packed into a solid pellet or artificial "embryo."

Upper Right - Within six hours the cells have smoothed the outer surface of the pellet ("embryo") which is still solid.

Lower Right - Within twenty hours the embryo has formed into a trilaminar hollow sphere. Cell loss occurs from surface layer.

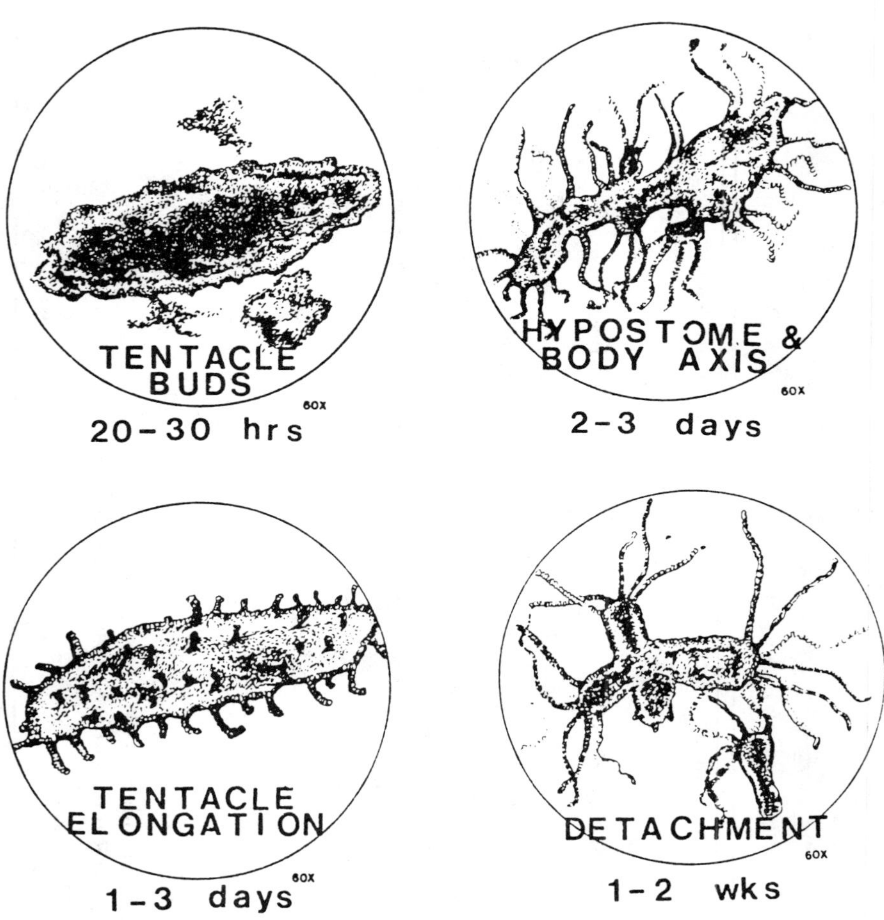

FIGURE 2   Diagramatic representation of regenerating **Hydra attenuata.**

Upper Left - By thirty hours small elevations appear indicating the initial differentiation of tentacles. Cells loss continues at reduced rate.

Lower Left - The tentacle buds elongate for the next 24 hours without obvious further development elsewhere in the embryo.

Upper Right - During the third day hypostomes appear and the tentacles become organized circumferentially around them. The number around each hypostome is brought to 6 by formation of new tentacles or regression of preexisting excess tentacles, depending on the local situation.

Lower Right - A body axis forms below each hypostome and by the end of a week the newly formed polyps begin to detach and live independently.

TABLE II

Effects of test substances on adult and artificial embryos of *Hydra attenuata*.

Lowest Toxic Concentration (μg/ml)

TEST MATERIAL	"EMBRYONIC"	"ADULT"	RATIO*
Actinomycin D	5	50	10
Aspirin	375	500	1.3
Dimethyl sulfoxide	10	20	2
Isoniazed (non-acetylated)	1	500	500
Lithium carbonate	40	80	2.0
Lithium chloride	50	90	1.8

*The larger the number is, the greater is the vulnerability of developmental events to the action of the material tested. Ratios within the same order of magnitude should not be considered as differing.

TABLE III

Effects* of test substances on *in utero* and adult rodents.

TEST SUBSTANCE	SPECIES & ROUTE	SOME COMPARABLE TOXIC DOSE "EMBRYONIC"	(mg/kg) "ADULT"	RATIO
Actinomycin D	mouse i.p./i.v.	0.14	0.67	4.8
Aspirin	rat i.p.	250	420	1.7
Dimethyl Sulfoxide	rat i.p.	8000	13000	1.6
	rat orl	5000	19700	3.4
Lithium carbonate	mouse orl	3000	531	5.6
Lithium chloride	rat i.p.	190	514	2.7
Isoniazid (non-acetylated)	rat orl	14	650	46

*For effects on developing and adult rodents to be compared, the species, route and duration of treatment as well as stain and observational level need to be similar.

ly, so the rose bush assay is invalid.

The simplified Segment II, the limb bud culture system and Hydra may have potential for identifying substances of marked potential for disrupting developmental events in the absence of adult toxicity and this is the bottom line of detecting potential teratogenic hazards. One additional system (1) should be mentioned because it also has possibilities. The system has not begun vigorous testing but such insects and other presumably primitive forms and their embryos should be examined carefully. At the level of their basic developmental biology they are not to be considered markedly different from any other developing system as regards the developmental phenomena employed during embryogenesis. An example of this would be that a substance disrupting cytoskeleton formation or function would preclude cell migrations in the embryo of each species and, if this were the mechanism of action of that substance, then abnormal ontogenesis will occur.

Since I have already taken the view that there is not much to be learned by looking at the positive characteristics of prescreens, I will point out that there may be great value in examining the other side of the coin. There are several items to be examined carefully in evaluating any prescreen and some of these are listed in Table 4.

TABLE IV

Considerations for evaluating the validity of teratology prescreens.

1. Inappropriately labeled substances.
2. Incomplete referencing.
3. Selective choice of compounds.
4. Yes/No answers or designations.
5. Selective choice of doses.
6. Need for prior information.
7. Dose response relationships.
8. Do data really recapitulate.
9. If the substance tested had been unknown, would the system have accurately predicted the general conclusions possible from more complex studies.

Accurate identification of substances as to their known level of developmental hazard potential is essential. It should be carefully determined whether or not the substances listed as 'non-teratogens' are actually established as being incapable of disrupting development. If one were to say that chloroform has no teratogenic capability and that a particular prescreen appropriately recapitulates this observation, it could be referenced accurately to the literature. The reference would be accurate in all regards. The problem would be that a subsequent reference establishes that chloroform is indeed capable of producing terata. In this manner the test system has not accurately predicted, but has given a false negative.

Selectivity in the mammalian species and route of administration chosen for comparison of data between mammals and the prescreening system can occur. Injection of the test material may give one type response, while another author may report results with an entirely different outcome just because a different route of administration was employed. In order to be considered valid a prescreen must account for this type of event in addition to the more obvious interspecies differences, etc., so very familiar to us all.

Selective choice of compounds could occur inadvertently and cause an investigator to inadvertently participate in a self-fulfilling prophecy such that the compounds would have been accurately identified for teratogenic potential even by a plastic rose bush. A buzzword here is 'variety' - test a wide variety of chemical types. This sounds good and is advisable, but of itself provides no assurances that the system has had an adequate test. This is because within each of a variety of chemical classifications or types one could inadvertently pick the single example from that class which the particular prescreening system will accurately identify as being or not being a potential developmental hazard.

Suspicions are aroused by a system purporting to identify substances as teratogenically black or white. If thalidomide, Vitamin A, vinblastin, and aspirin are all called teratogens by a prescreen, this is accurate but such simple identifications demonstrate the system as not applicable to the real world. The degree of teratogenic potential needs to be established by the prescreen. Similarly to declare a substance a 'non-teratogen' countermands Karnofsky's law and so far that has not been possible. That is, if enough of a substance is administered to some species, a dose will be found which can cause disruptive effects on some aspect of development. In the four chemicals just listed two are teratogenic hazards by everyone's experience while the other two are eliminated from consideration by the experienced toxicologist because the doses required for teratogenesis are too close or are synonymous with the adult toxic doses for those same substances. That is, they are coeffective teratogens in that they are toxic to both the adult and the conceptus at the same general dose level.

If different compounds are tested at different doses based on preexisting data, then the system has a problem. This may not be insurmountable but it does need recognition by the authors because a prescreen ultimately must function in the world of no, or very minimal, prior data and should be able to function even for an effluent compound or complex mixture of unknown composition.

SUMMARY

A prescreen should be able to identify a potential teratogenic hazard in the absence of prior information.

Dose response relationships should be generated by the system as a part of its cause and effect validation. A basic premise of toxicology is a dose response relationship. This is generally true whether one is scientifically examining water injection for avoiding major earthquakes or determining whether or not TCDD needs regulation on the basis of posing a threat to the conceptus.

A prescreen needs to accurately recapitulate the preexisting data and do it in a manner that allows retrospective prediction of what the teratogenic dose was in a standard evaluation. It should do this rapidly and at low cost.

Acknowledgment

The technical assistance of Regina M. Gorman, Bradley E.G. Gable and Mindy E. George is gratefully acknowledged.

REFERENCES

1. Bournias-Vardiabasis, N., R.L. Teplitz, and R.L. Seecof 1980 An in vitro assay of teratogenesis. Teratology 21:29A.
2. Chatot, C.L., N.W. Klein, J. Piatek, and L.J. Pierro 1980 Successful culture of rat embryos on human serum: use in detecting teratogens. Science 207:1471-1473.
3. Chernof, N. and R.J. Kavlock 1980 A potential *in vivo* screen for the determination of teratogenic effects in mammals. Teratology *21:* 33A-34A.
4. Gierer, A.B., H. Bode, C.N. David, K. Flick, G. Hansmann, H. Schaller, and E. Trenkner 1972 Regeneration of hydra from reaggregating cells. Nature New Biol. 239: 98-105.
5. Johnson, E.M. 1980a Screening for teratogenic potential: are we asking the proper question. Teratology *21:* 259.
6. Johnson, E.M. 1980b A subvertebrate system for rapid determination of potential teratogenic hazards. J. Environ. Path. Tox. *4:*
7. Johnson, 1981 Screening for teratogenic hazards: nature of the problem. Ann. Rev. Pharm. Tox. *21:* 415:429. Annual Reviews Inc., Palo Alto (in press).
8. Karnofsky, D.A. 1965 Mechanisms of action of certain growth-inhibiting drugs. In: *Teratology: Principles and Techniques.* Ed. by J.G. Wilson and J. Warkany. Univ. of Chicago Press. Chapter 8.
9. Kochhar, D.M. and M.B. Aydelotte 1974 Susceptible stages and abnormal morphogenesis in the developing mouse limb, analyzed in organ culture after transplacental exposure to vitamin A (retinoic acid). J. Embryol. exp. Morph. *31:* 721-734.
10. Kochar, D.M. 1975 The use of in vitro procedures in teratology. Teratology, *11:* 273-288.
11. Kochhar, D.M. 1981 Embryo explants and organ cultures in screening

of chemicals for teratogenic effects. Chapter 10 in *Developmental Toxicity*. Raven Press, N.Y. (in press).

12. Russel, L.B. 1979 Sensitivity pattern for the induction of homeotic shifts in a favorable strain of mice. Teratology *20:* 115-126.

13. Russel, L.B. 1980 Utilization of critical periods during development to study the effects of low levels of environmental agents. Proceedings of the Rochester Symposium. Plenum Press (in press).

14. Schardein, J.L. 1976 *Drugs as Teratogens*. CRC Press, Cleveland.

15. Shepard, T.H. 1980 *Catalog of Teratogenic Agents*. Third Edition, The Johns Hopkins Univ. Press, Baltimore.

16. Walton, B.T. 1981 Chemical impurity produces extra compound eyes and heads in crickets. Science *212:* 51-53.

SECTION II

ORNL/EIS-197
EPA-600/9-82-001

Contract No. W-7405-eng-26

ASSESSMENT OF RISKS TO HUMAN REPRODUCTION AND TO DEVELOPMENT OF THE HUMAN CONCEPTUS FROM EXPOSURE TO ENVIRONMENTAL SUBSTANCES

Proceedings of U.S. Environmental Protection Agency—
Sponsored Conferences:

October 1–3, 1980, Atlanta, Georgia,
and
December 7–10, 1980, St. Louis, Missouri

Wayne M. Galbraith, Ph.D.
Peter Voytek, Ph.D.
Office of Research and Development
U.S. Environmental Protection Agency
Washington, D.C. 20460

and

Michael G. Ryon, M.S.
Chemical Effects Information Center
Information Center Complex
Information Division
Oak Ridge National Laboratory
Oak Ridge, Tennessee 37830

Work sponsored by the U.S. Environmental Protection Agency,
Washington, D.C., under Interagency Agreements
No. 80-D-X1011 and No. 81-D-X0453

OAK RIDGE NATIONAL LABORATORY
Oak Ridge, Tennessee 37830
operated by
UNION CARBIDE CORPORATION
for the
DEPARTMENT OF ENERGY

CONTENTS

Tables   x
Acknowledgments   xi
CHAPTER 1
Introduction   1
CHAPTER 2
Female Reproduction   3
  General Reproductive Toxicity Screen   3
  Qualitative Reproductive Toxicity Tests   5
    Estrogen agonist-antagonist   5
    Androgen agonist-antagonist   5
    Nonsteroidal toxicant screening tests   6
    Computerized integrated data base   6
  Quantitative Reproductive Toxicity Tests   6
  Risk Assessment   7
  Research Needed   9
    Qualitative reproductive toxicity tests   9
    Quantitative reproductive toxicity tests   10
    Specific recommendations   10
    Extrapolation of animal data to humans   11
References   12
Appendix   13
Details of Test Protocols and Glossary of Terms for
  Female Risk Assessments   13
Description and Discussion of Tests Useful in Assessing
  Risk to the Female Reproductive System   13
  Qualitative Reproductive Toxicity Tests   13
    Estrogen agonist-antagonist   13
    Androgen agonist-antagonist   14
    Nonsteroidal toxicant screening tests   14
  Quantitative Reproductive Toxicity Tests   18
    Estrogen agonist-antagonist   18
    Androgen agonist-antagonist   19
  Hypothalamic-Pituitary Function Tests   21
    Assay of agents that stimulate the release of
      gonadotropins from cells of the anterior
      pituitary gland   21

Assays of agents that inhibit the release of
gonadotropins from cells of the anterior
pituitary gland 22
Assay of an agent that inhibits the release of
prolactin from cells of the anterior pituitary
gland 23
Assay of an agent that inhibits the release of
prolactin from pituitary cells 23
Assay of the activity of an agent that alters the
secretion of dopamine by hypothalamic
neurons 24
Assay of the activity of an agent that alters the
secretion of norepinephrine by hypothalamic
neurons 24
Assay of the activity of an agent that alters the
secretion of GnRH 24
Assay of the activity of an agent that alters the
secretion of hypothalamic opioid peptides 25
Blood flow of the hypothalamic-hypophysial system . . 25
Sexual behavior tests 25
Ovarian Toxicity 27
Oocyte and follicle toxicity 27
Inhibition of steroidogenesis 28
References 34
Glossary of Terms Used in Female Reproduction 37
CHAPTER 3
Considerations in Evaluating Risk to Male
Reproduction 41
Introduction 41
Aspects of the Problem 42
Selection of an Animal Model 43
Tests for Evaluating Reproductive Damage 46
Evaluation of Reproductive Damage in Exposed or
Potentially Exposed Men 52
General 52
Surveillance studies 52
Study of men with known toxic exposure 53
Additional comment on human testing procedures . . . 54
Assessment of risk to men 55
Protocols for Testing Compounds with Animal Models . . 57
Test 1 — initial screen 57
Test 2 — dose response curve 57
Test 3 — recovery study 59

Research Needed 60
References 63
Appendix 69
Details of Test Protocols and Glossary of Terms for
   Male Risk Assessment 69
  Description and Discussion of Tests Useful in
   Animal Models or Man 69
  Body weight 69
  Testicular Characteristics 69
   Testis size in situ 69
   Testis weight 70
   Spermatid reserves 70
   Histopathological analysis of testes 71
   Counts of preleptotene or leptotene
    spermatocytes 72
  Epididymal Characteristics 72
   Weight of distal half of epididymis 72
   Number of sperm in the distal half of
    epididymis 72
   Motility of sperm from the distal end 72
   Gross morphology of spermatozoa from the
    distal end 73
   Detailed morphology of spermatozoa from the
    distal end 73
  Accessory Sex Gland Characteristics 73
  Seminal Analysis 73
   General aspects of seminal analysis 73
   Volume 75
   Seminal plasma constituents 75
   Spermatozoal concentration 76
   Total sperm per ejaculate 76
   Sperm motility 77
   Spermatozoal morphology 78
   Ejaculated sperm as an *in vitro* test system 79
  Assessment of Male Reproductive Toxicity Using
   Endocrinological Methods 79
   General 79
   Hormone assay and application 80
  Examination of Known Toxic Exposures 82
   Humans 82
   Animal models 83

Fertility Testing 84
   Tests available 84
   Usefulness 85
   Sensitivity 85
   Specificity 86
Sperm Nucleus Integrity 86
   Quinacrine staining for Y-chromosome
     aneuploidy 86
   Spermatozoal morphology 87
   Karyotyping of human spermatozoa by the
     denuded-hamster-egg technique 87
Dose Response 87
References 88
Glossary of Terms Used in Male Reproduction 93
CHAPTER 4
Current Status of, and Considerations for, Estimation
   of Risk to the Human Conceptus from
   Environmental Chemicals 99
Definition and Scope 99
Impact of Developmental Abnormalities on Humans . . . 99
Causes of Congenital Malformations 100
Qualitative Evaluation of Risk Potential 100
   Interspecies comparisons 100
   Dosing and mode of administration 101
   Placental transfer 102
   Pharmacokinetics and metabolism 103
   Mechanisms of action 103
Animal Studies 104
   Standard teratogenicity testing 104
   Functional teratogenicity testing 106
Short-Term Testing Procedures 107
   Prioritizing of chemicals for in-depth study 107
   Characteristics of short-term assays 108
   Potential short-term systems 109
Quantitative Risk Assessment 110
Priorities for Future Research in Teratology 112
References 113
CHAPTER 5
Other Considerations: Epidemiology, Pharmacokinetics,
   and Sexual Behavior 117
Epidemiology: Methods and Limitations 117
   Hypothesis generating studies 117

Analytic studies for formally testing hypotheses
and quantifying risks 118
Limitations 118
Possible data sources and useful approaches 120
Pharmacokinetics 121
Sexual Behavior 123
Introduction 123
Qualitative evaluation of risk potential 128
Animal studies 131
Assessment of human sexual behavior:
surveillance and epidemiological
studies 136
Priority areas for future research 139
References 141
Steering Committee 145
Participants 147
Reviewers 151
Index 153

TABLES

1. Reproductive Processes Potentially Susceptible
   to Reproductive Toxicants 8
2. Estrogen Agonist Screen 14
3. Time Table for Intergenerational Protocol to Evaluate
   Putative Toxicant Effects on Reproduction in Sexually
   Mature Animals 15
4. Compounds Tested for Oocyte/Follicle Toxicity in
   the Murine Assay 29
5. Agents That Inhibit Steroidogenesis 31
6. Features of Ovarian Cell Preparations, *In Vitro,*
   Potentially Useful in Xenobiotic Inhibition of
   Steroidogenesis 33
7. Criteria for Evaluation of Male Reproduction in
   Favored Animal Models and Man 44
8. Tests Considered Useful for Screening Toxic
   Compounds 47
9. Reasons for Rejection of Potential Evaluation
   Tests Considered by Male Reproductive
   Subgroup 49
10. Approximate Variation Between Animals for
    Suggested Test Criteria (CV) Coefficient of
    Variation (%) 50
11. Chronology of Conduct for Test with Animal
    Models 58
12. Some *In Vitro* Short-Term Systems Currently
    in Various Stages of Development 110

ACKNOWLEDGMENTS

This document resulted from discussions at two conference meetings sponsored by the U.S. Environmental Protection Agency (EPA). The first meeting took place in Atlanta, Georgia, October 1–3, 1980, and the second, in St. Louis, Missouri, December 7–10, 1980. The participants in this project are listed at the back of this document; their interest, scientific knowledge, and contributions of personal and professional time are largely responsible for the production of this report. The steering committee and the group chairmen contributed additionally by selecting participants, organizing subject agenda, and refining reports produced during the conferences. In particular, Drs. Richard Hoar and Marshall Johnson played major roles throughout the duration of the project. The final step involved external reviews, and the contributors to this process are also listed in the back of this report.

In addition to the input from the scientific community, efforts of the technical staff from Oak Ridge National Laboratory played a large role in the success of the project. Joy Simmons and Norma Callaham handled arrangements for hotel accommodations and equipment rental. Debra Ballard, Evelyn Daniel, Pat Hartman, Robert Ross, and John Smith provided word processing and logistical support for the participants during the conferences. Members of the Technical Publications Department, especially Pat Hartman and Donna Stokes, were responsible for typing, and John Getsi, for editing the drafts into finished form.

The U.S. EPA's Offices of Research and Development and of Pesticides and Toxic Substances and the Oak Ridge National Laboratory gratefully acknowledge the efforts of all those involved and thank them for assisting in this project.

Wayne Galbraith, U.S. EPA Co—Project Officer
Peter Voytek, U.S. EPA Co—Project Officer
Michael Ryon, ORNL Conference Coordinator

ACKNOWLEDGMENTS

CHAPTER 1

Peter Voytek
US Environmental Protection Agency
Washington, DC 20460

INTRODUCTION

The U.S. Environmental Protection Agency (EPA) has the legislative mandate to consider regulatory alternatives for chemicals that are causing or can cause a health hazard to man. Because the reproductive system contains some of the more sensitive targets of potentially hazardous agents whose impact on human populations may be immediate, toxicity to the reproductive system and the conceptus is of emerging scientific and social interest. As a result of this interest, the Offices of Health Research and of Health and Environmental Assessment within the Office of Research and Development sponsored a conference to produce a technical document on the current status of risk assessment methodologies for teratogenic and other reproductive effects. The conference brought together scientists knowledgeable in reproductive biology and teratology to discuss techniques and concepts pertinent to developing risk assessment methodologies.

Conference participants were selected based on their expertise in the various disciplines of reproductive biology, statistics, pharmacokinetics, endocrinology, epidemiology, and sexual behavioral toxicology. Draft copies of the report were sent to numerous scientists in academia and the private sector for peer review, and their comments were used by the members of the conference to modify the final document.

The document is divided into three main subject areas: assessment of toxicity to female reproduction, assessment of toxicity to male reproduction, and assessment of toxicity to the conceptus. There are three supplemental parts: pharmacokinetics and epidemiologic considerations, which are common to all toxicological assessments, and a special section on the behavioral aspects of sexual development.

The specific areas addressed in this report are the potential adverse effects on the female and male reproductive systems as well as adverse effects on the developing conceptus. A broad range of problems and effects are discussed, including infertility, early resorption of the conceptus, and possible behavioral disorders produced by subtle changes in the biochemical environment of the fetus.

The report also provides suggestions for improvement in standard toxicological protocols for evaluation of reproductive risks, identifies new concepts and procedures that can be immediately applicable, and designates those that need further expansion and development through research. Included is a discussion on the predictive ability of the tests in estimating risk.

The information in this document will be of value not only to scientists conducting experiments on the effects of chemical agents on the reproductive system, but also to those that need to assess the results from such studies. Thus many tests discussed herein may currently be inappropriate, economically or technically, for regulatory use, but are included to provide necessary and useful background information for evaluating data.

In assessing human risks from exposure to potentially toxic chemicals, many considerations should be addressed, such as severity and reversibility/irreversibility of the effect, existence of threshold or nonthreshold levels, dose-response relationships, sensitivity of the toxicological response evaluated, and predictive ability of animal studies to determine the risk to humans. Attempts have been made in this document to address these considerations.

CHAPTER 2
FEMALE REPRODUCTION

James H. Clark
Baylor College of Medicine
Houston, TX 77030

Risk assessment for toxicants that alter reproduction in females involves two separate but equally critical tasks. These are assessment of reproductive parameters in laboratory animals to identify compounds that are prospective reproductive toxicants and continuous epidemiologic surveillance of normal human reproductive characteristics to identify their prevalence, trends, and geographical differences and their potential modification by environmental events. An approach to the evaluation of epidemiologic data is provided in Chapter 5.

The problem of risk assessment has been approached by proposing an animal screening system for qualitative and quantitative analysis of reproductive toxicants. This system is coupled to an integrated data base that serves as a mechanism for the analysis of structure-function relationships of potential toxins. These testing systems form a comprehensive screening scheme that should serve to detect reproductive toxins and provide a foundation for risk assessment. In addition, such a system will serve as a repository of information into which continued input should expand our understanding of risk assessment and reproductive toxicology.

General Reproductive Toxicity Screen

We propose that the stepwise scheme shown in Fig. 1 be followed in an attempt to identify compounds presently in the environment for which there is epidemiologic evidence of adverse reproductive effect and to identify new compounds that may be disseminated into the environment. At the first level, a compound should be tested by the laboratory procedures described below. The standard acute, subacute, and subchronic toxicological testing protocols do not incorporate procedures for detection of reproductive effects, and therefore the following screening procedures were specifically designed for this purpose. If the result of any screening test is positive, the compound must be evaluated by the quantitative risk assessment procedures. If the screening tests are all negative, the compound

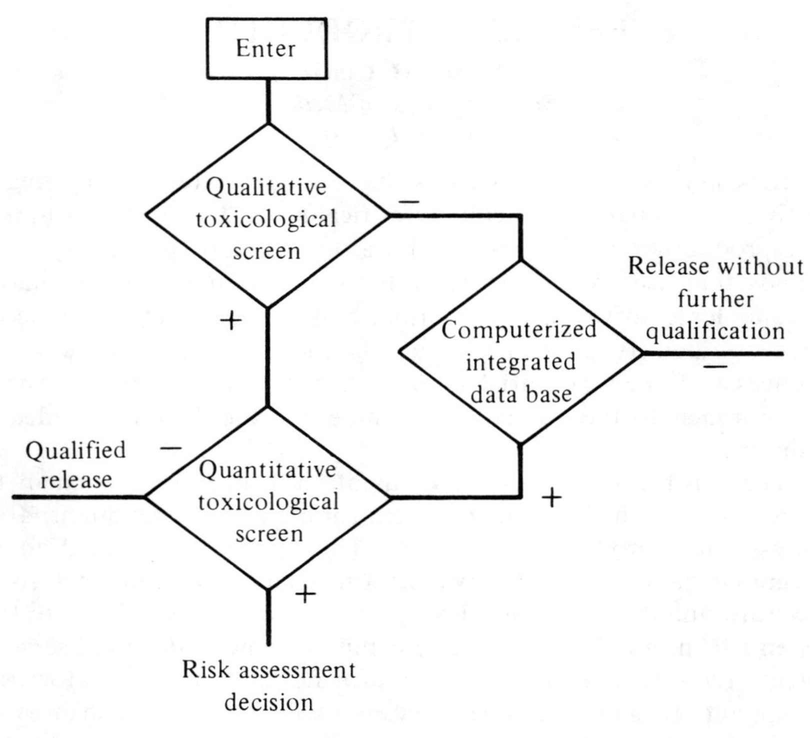

Figure 1 — Reproductive toxicity assessment prospective evaluation.

must then be compared by the computerized integrated data base for structural relationships and/or similarities in the probable pharmaco-kinetics witn other compounds known to affect the reproductive system. An examination of the potential degradation products of the compound, using a computer model analysis of its chemical structure, might also prove useful. If the compound is found to have a structural or functional similarity to known active agents, it must undergo the quantitative risk assessment procedures. If no such affinity is found (and the qualitative screen is entirely negative), the compound can be released into the environment without further testing.

If a compound that enters the quantitative risk assessment procedures is found to be without activity ("false positive" in screens or in search for structural affinity), it can be given qualified approval. That is, its use must be restricted and accompanied by appropriately directed epidemiologic surveillance.

If a compound that enters the quantitative risk assessment procedure is positive, the risk for humans should be estimated, insofar as possible. This information must be weighed and the decision made about whether the compound can be released at all and if so, with what restrictions.

Qualitative Reproductive Toxicity Tests

Estrogen agonist—antagonist

Estrogens mediate, integrate, and modulate interaction of the hypothalamic-hypophyseal-gonadal axis and, as such, are important hormones in the control of reproduction. Exposure to exogenous estrogens is known to have deleterious effects on reproductive potential (1). For predicting the estrogenicity of environmental chemicals, a series of simple screening tests are proposed. These include (a) time of vaginal opening in the neonatal rat, (b) uterine epithelial cellular hypertrophy, and (c) estrogen-receptor-binding analysis. These tests have been chosen because of their sensitivity to estrogenlike substances and the close correlations that exist between these estrogenic responses and subsequent abnormal reproductive capacity. For details of the test procedures, see the Appendix to this chapter.

The tests cited above can be used to detect estrogen toxicants; however, they could also be used to classify estrogen agonist-antagonist. Generally, a decreased response in the tests would indicate an antagonistic effect, whereas an increased response would indicate an agonistic effect. Such a classification scheme, which would require extension and expansion of the tests cited, could form the basis for a structure-function data bank for the prediction of estrogenic toxicity.

Androgen agonist—antagonist

Androgenic substances are known to cause infertility in female animals, and their effects on the human fetus are well known. Exposure to androgens during pregnancy causes masculinization of female fetuses and various physiological and behavioral problems in the adult. Androgenic compounds can be assessed by their capacity to stimulate weight increases in the ventral prostate and seminal vesicles of the intact immature male rat or mouse. This assay is acceptable and practical for predicting androgenic effects (agonistic and/or antagonistic) in humans.

It is important to determine whether a potential toxicant influences development or reproductive capabilities. For this purpose, determining responses of newborn rats following exposure to suitable doses of the potential toxicant provides a multifactorial assay. Similarly, screening tests (e.g., testosterone blood levels or accessory sex gland weight) for androgen antagonists are also available. More sensitive tests for androgen agonists/antagonists are described in the quantitative section of Female Reproduction and in the Appendix to this chapter.

Nonsteroidal toxicant screening tests

The preceding tests will detect estrogenic and androgenic toxicants. For testing of substances other than these two classes of compounds, a multigenerational protocol is proposed. This protocol is designed to evaluate (a) adult female conceptive ability with initial exposure to the agent occurring near puberty, (b) the effect on pregnancy, (c) potential transmission during lactation, and (d) reproductive performance of the second generation. As a standard approach to the testing of potential reproductive toxicants, these tests will detect substances that interfere with reproduction at various levels of biological organization. (For details see the Appendix.)

Computerized integrated data base

The computerized integrated data base should include all known structure-function relationships for reproductive toxicants. With such a data base it would be possible to construct reproductive toxicant profiles (activity profiles) that would predict the potential activity of putative toxicants. Admittedly, such a scheme has shortcomings and prediction will not be perfect. However, if at some future date sufficient information were available in the data base, it could prove to be most useful and time saving.

Quantitative Reproductive Toxicity Tests

The screening tests outlined in the previous section are designed to identify compounds that may represent reproductive hazards.

Once a compound is found to have either a reproductive effect in the qualitative screen or a structural relationship with known active agents in the computerized-integrated-data-base screen, a more detailed quantitative evaluation is mandatory. This process will vary substantially, depending on the type of effects seen in the qualitative screen or the characteristics of the known toxicant to which it appears similar. These tests for quantitative assessment, which are presented in detail in the Appendix to this chapter, can be used to determine site or locus of action of these xenobiotics. It is important to recognize that some xenobiotics may act at more than one site and by more than one mechanism. Ultimately, these specific assays have the potential to determine risk of exposures. In this document an attempt is made to provide an interface between female reproductive biology and toxicology.

Risk Assessment

Assessment of risks to the female reproductive system from environmental sources will have to involve a broad class of potentially affected processes, organs, and structures obtained from human exposure and relevant laboratory results. The reversibility of effects needs to be considered carefully. The applicability of the available information to potential environmental exposure will need to be considered. The magnitude of human risk for reproductive toxicity may be modulated by such diverse factors as distribution of the compound in the environment, patterns of use or exposure, persistence in the biosphere, concentration in the food chain, and age-dependent changes in sensitivity.

Risk assessment will require a knowledge of pertinent factors related to the reproductive process and of relationships of specialized laboratory results to these factors. If a compound demonstrates a reproductive effect in any mammalian species, this observation indicates that some concern about actual human exposure to the agent is justified. Positive results in a number of laboratory tests, which by themselves may be only suggestive of harm, will be important in evaluating potentially detrimental effects.

Substantial modifications in any of the subsystems given in Table 1 are known to be serious and should be avoided. Future testing may indicate relationships between these subsystems and other laboratory testing. Risk assessment for female reproduction requires the establishment of assays relevant to these reproductive processes and the validation of these assays in identifying substances actually toxic to human reproduction. The assays should be shown

TABLE 1 Reproductive Processes Potentially
Susceptible to Reproductive Toxicants

	Nonpregnant	Pregnant
Vulva/Vagina	Virilization Adenosis	
Cervix	Structural abnormalities Mucus production and/or quality	Incompetence

Uterus	Luminal fluid
	Structural malformations
	Dysfunctional bleeding
	Dyssynergia
	Deficient pseudodecidual
	  response
		Untimely parturition
		Dysfunctional labor
		Uterine blood flow
		Gestational trophoblastic
		  disease
		Deficient decidual response

Fallopian Tube	Gamete transport fluid	Zygote transport Ectopic pregnancy

Ovary	Decreased number of oocytes
	Increased rate of follicular
	  atresia
	Follicular: steroidogenesis
	         maturation
	         rupture
	         fluid quality
	Oocyte maturation
	Luteal function
	Chronic anovulation
		Luteal function

Breast	Supernumerary mammary glands
	Galactorrhea
	Nongalactorrheic discharge
	Gynecomastia
		Lactational transport of
		  toxicants
		Lactation: composition
		  capability

Placenta		Transplacental transport of toxicants Hydatidiform mole Enzymatic activities

Pituitary	Hyperprolactinemia
	Hypoprolactinemia
	Altered synthesis and
	  release of trophic
	  hormones	

Hypothalamus	Altered synthesis and
	  release of neurotransmitters,
	  neuromodulators, and
	  neurohormones	

Liver	Metabolism Binding protein synthesis	Metabolism Binding protein synthesis
Adrenal	Steroidogenesis	Steroidogenesis
Behavior	Sexual behavior	Maternal behavior
Reproductive lifespan	Puberty Menopause	

to be relevant in the species used, especially any assays adapted from human assays, and should avoid complications such as those resulting from diurnal variations in hormone level. The results from these studies may indicate other areas where regulation will be necessary.

It is generally felt that when dose-response relationships are observed, lowering exposure will cause less harm when the compound is xenobiotic, unless evidence to the contrary exists. Consideration could be given to using safety factors to establish acceptable exposure levels in situations where harm can reasonably be expected and the exposure cannot reasonably be avoided.

Research Needed

Qualitative reproductive toxicity tests

The scheme for the detection of reproductive toxicity discussed earlier and diagramed in Fig. 1 proposes further investigation in several research areas. One such area is that of structure-function relationships, which are not well understood at the present time. No one would have predicted from the structure of kepone that it would bind to the estrogen receptors and stimulate estrogenic responses. Obviously, much needs to be learned about what constitutes an estrogenic molecule. However, kepone would have been detected as an estrogen by the above tests, and indeed, had more been known about structure-function relationships, it might have been suspected before any tests were performed.

The establishment of reproductive-toxicological profiles and structure-function prediction models has just begun. Much basic information is required before such a system can be realized. Therefore, a strong recommendation is that basic research in reproductive toxicity be supported, with a major emphasis on establishing such models.

An important component of the qualitative reproductive toxicity screen is the computerized integrated data base (see Fig. 1). With such a data base, it should be possible to predict the potential toxicity of putative toxicants. That such a predictive scheme has its faults is well recognized; however, further efforts to realize the potential of such a system should not be discouraged on account of these. In theory, when sufficient information is available concerning structure-function relationships of toxicants, such a prediction scheme may decrease the need for extensive animal testing. For this reason it is recommended that further attempts to establish and validate such a data base be made and also that arrangements be made to update continuously such a facility, with the ultimate intent of perfecting predictive potential.

Quantitative reproductive toxicity tests

The recommendations concerning the qualitative tests also apply to the proposed quantitative tests. The information gained from the quantitative tests extend and interplay with the results obtained from the qualitative tests. Therefore, it is recommended that information gained from the quantitative tests be integrated with that obtained from the qualitative tests to permit an even greater understanding of structure-function relationships.

Specific recommendations

1. The relationship between cellular receptors for toxicants and their mechanism of action should be explored further. Such information can be fed directly into a structure-function data bank such as the computerized integrated data base.

2. More work is obviously needed regarding masculinization of the female, an important problem in reproductive toxicity evaluations. Few data are available on dose responses of these effects, and fewer data exist regarding inhibition (antagonism) of the alteration. Further, extrapolation of these data to humans is not possible, because subhuman primates and humans do not sustain substantial defects of ovulation, whereas sexual behavior is altered. Information presently available is insufficient for determining whether this discrepancy is due to the fetal age at which treatment was administered or to actual differences in sensitivities.

3. *In vitro* model systems are needed (in many areas) for the assessment of reproductive toxicants. For example, model systems for the secretion of gonadotropins by the pituitary cells can be used to study toxicants that influence this process. Currently, almost nothing is known about such model systems, and their value for predicting toxicity is potentially great.

Another important *in vitro* model system in need of development is that of inhibition of steroidogenesis. Although this system has been well characterized for many inhibitors (see the Appendix to this chapter), it has not been exploited for its potential as a test system for toxicants. Continued work and support will be needed to develop these model systems and to relate the information obtained to that gathered from *in vivo* studies.

4. Because little is known about the effects of neuroactive substances such as dopamine and norephinephrine on the hypothalamic-hypophysial complex and about the effects of toxicants on this system, research support should be allocated to this important field, both for the development of new methods and for studies on the mechanism of action.

5. Support is recommended for development of models and research on basic mechanisms in behavioral toxicology, an area in which many unknowns exist regarding reproductive toxicity (see the Appendix).

6. Much work is needed in oocyte toxicity, an obviously important area of concern in which there are incompletely understood age, strain, and species differences in sensitivity of ovotoxicity. For example, preovulatory and growing follicles are most sensitive to toxicity in humans, whereas resting follicles are most sensitive in mice. Similarly, significant differences in sensitivity to oocyte destruction exist between mice and rats. However, evidence from studies exploring the effects of antitumor agents on humans and experimental animals suggests that a compound demonstrated to be ovotoxic in rodents will also be ovotoxic in humans.

Extrapolation of animal data to humans

The primary goal of risk assessment for environmental agents is directed toward adverse effect(s) (injury) in human individuals or human populations. In most cases data are available only in animal model systems; hence it is necessary to extrapolate these findings to anticipated changes in humans. Although extrapolations may be possible, it should be noted that our current understanding of the relationships between hormone exposure and toxic outcomes is not optimal. The following discussion is included to illustrate this point.

An increased rate of vascular disease in women taking oral contraceptive pills has been reported by several investigators (see Kay [2] for review). This has been generally attributed to the estrogenic component of the pill and at first may seem to represent a source of data concerning estrogen levels and toxic effects. However, as Kay (2) points out, the progesterone content of the pill, not the estrogen content, is correlated with increased incidence of vascular disease. Progesterone has also been shown to decrease high-density lipoprotein (HDL) cholesterol, an event associated with increased risk of arteriosclerosis. Estrogens increase HDL cholesterol and therefore would be expected to decrease the incidence of vascular disease. Obviously, predicting risks based on estrogen levels in women taking the pill requires further consideration.

This example points out the need for more research at all levels, from biochemical to epidemiological, and emphasizes the requirement for more data before meaningful extrapolations can be made for risk assessment in humans.

REFERENCES

1. McLachlan, J.: Estrogens in the environment. Elsevier/North Holland: New York; 419 pp., 1980.
2. Kay, C. R.: The happiness pill? J. R. Coll. Gen. Pract. 30: 8–19, 1980.

APPENDIX

DETAILS OF TEST PROTOCOLS AND GLOSSARY OF TERMS FOR FEMALE RISK ASSESSMENTS

I. DESCRIPTION AND DISCUSSION OF TESTS USEFUL IN ASSESSING RISK TO THE FEMALE REPRODUCTIVE SYSTEM

Qualitative Reproductive Toxicity Tests

Estrogen agonist—antagonist

Time of vaginal opening in the neonatal rat. Rats are injected on days 1, 3, and 5 of postnatal life, and the time of vaginal opening is noted. Estrogen agonists such as diethylstilbestrol (DES), clomiphene, and tamoxifen are known to cause early maturation of vaginal development (1–3), and this test serves as a sensitive indication of such activity. The general protocol for this test for estrogen agonist is shown in Table 2.

Uterine epithelial cellular hypertrophy. Neonatal rats are treated as described in Table 2, and the uteri are taken on day 7 for histological examination. Epithelial cell growth is an excellent indicator of estrogenicity and will detect compounds, such as clomiphene, which exhibit differential cell stimulation (4). Kepone, DES, dichlorodiphenyltrichloroethane (DDT), and zearlenone have been shown to be either active in this test or very likely active because of their known ability to stimulate uterine growth (4, 5).

The above tests, requiring a minimal number of animals, are simple and reliable. These tests are used routinely in many laboratories and are quite sensitive to estrogenic compounds (μg/kg).

Estrogen-receptor-binding analysis. Uteri obtained from 7-day-old rats which have been treated as described above are examined for nuclear binding of the estrogen receptor by the nuclear exchange assay (4). In the same tissues the quantity of cytoplasmic estrogen receptor can also be determined. This test gives a measure of the

TABLE 2   Estrogen Agonist Screen

Age (days)	Treatment of female rats
0	Birth
4	Beginning of daily dosing for 4 days
7	Sacrifice
	Assays:
	1 – uterine weight
	2 – endometrial histology
	3 – estrogen receptor assays
	4 – vaginal opening[a]

[a]Vaginal opening may occur by day 7; however, a longer time interval after birth may be required (up to 20 days).

ability of a toxicant to bind to estrogen receptor *in vivo* and to cause nuclear accumulation of the receptor-ligand complex. Classical estrogens such as estradiol and DES are known to perform this function, which is presumed to be an obligatory step in the mechanism of action of estrogens. Kepone, DDT, and zearlenone bind to the estrogen receptors, cause nuclear accumulation, and stimulate uterine growth (3, 5 6). Therefore, these compounds are likely to be active in the other tests for estrogenicity and will make excellent reference compounds for testing the model.

Androgen agonist–antagonist

These tests are standard and require no further explanation.

Nonsteroidal toxicant screening tests

This protocol is designed to evaluate: (a) ability of the adult female to conceive with the initial exposure to the agent near puberty (P-generation, Table 3); (b) the effect on pregnancy (live birth index of F_1, F_1^1, F_2, F_2^1 generations); (c) potential transmission during lactation (survival index of F_1 and F_2 generations); and (d) reproductive performance of the second generation (live birth index of F_1 and F_2 generations). Part of the P_1 generation (P_1^1) is mated again at the time of postpartum estrus, because at that time mating behavior, ovulation, implantation, and fetal resorption are more sensitive to environmental disruption than they are during mating at a cycling estrus.

TABLE 3 Time Table for Intergenerational Protocol to Evaluate Putative Toxicant Effects on Reproduction in Sexually Mature Animals

Approximate Time (weeks)	Parent (P_1) Generation (female)	F_1 Offspring	F_2 Offspring
0	P_1 – born		
6	P_1 – dosing begins		
10	P_1 – mated		
~13	P_1 – bears and suckles F_1 litter (dosing continued)		
	P_1^a – postpartum mated (dosing continued)		
~16	P_1^1 – bears F_1^1 litter[b]	F_1 – weaned, dosing begins	
~23		F_1 – mated first time (females)	
~26		F_1 – bears first litter (F_2)	
~29			F_2 – weaned, sacrificed
~40		F_1 – mated second time	
~43		F_1 – bears second litter $(F_2^1)^c$	

[a]Represents that portion of the P_1 generation that is mated at postpartum estrus.
[b]The F_1^1 litter is used as a check for the reproductive efficiency of the P_1^1 postpartum mating.
[c]The F_2^1 litter is used as a check for the reproductive efficiency of the second F_1 mating.

The age at which the animals are mated is a major procedural factor that can influence the fertility test results in the F_1 and F_2 generations. Toxicants, particularly those that possess steroidal activity, will diminish the success of pregnancy and number of offspring of older females but not those of younger females. Thus, while testing at earlier ages is more economical, it might yield false negative results. Therefore, a portion of the F_1 generation should be examined for ovarian cyclicity and fertility at approximately six months of age (live birth index of $F_{\frac{1}{2}}$ generation).

Experimental, vehicle control, and positive control (use of a known toxicant to verify the system) groups should be utilized with at least 20 animals per group. Selecting the agent to be used as a positive control will be arbitrary, and species or strain differences may complicate the choice. Despite these drawbacks, inclusion of a positive control that most appropriately parallels the test compound would seem mandatory for validation of the test system. The entire protocol need not be completed if adverse effects are demonstrated early in the protocol (i.e., live birth index of the F_1 generation).

The maximum tolerated dose should be used. Other dose levels may be included if dose response information is needed. Route of administration should be in food or water to avoid handling pregnant and lactating females, which may result in stress independent of that potentially caused by the agent being tested. This may complicate quantification of the ingested dose but ensures continuous dosing of the F_1 generation during weaning. Other routes of exposure (e.g., gavage or parenteral administration) may be used if the test protocol can be modified to avoid any interfering stress. Dosing begins at six weeks of age of the P_1 generation and continues until the end of the protocol. Body weights should be recorded weekly for all animals in the P_1 and F_1 generations as well as pup weights in the F_1, F_1^1, F_2, and $F_{\frac{1}{2}}$ offspring.

P_1 females are mated with untreated males of proven fertility at ten weeks of age in a one-to-one sex ratio. Successful mating is determined by finding a copulation plug and presence of sperm in the vaginal smear. These same females are then mated again at the time of postpartum estrus, 8—10 hours after giving birth. Twenty females from the F_1 generation (the offspring resulting from the first mating), are randomly selected and mated with untreated males of proven fertility at ten weeks of age. The offspring of postpartum mating (F_1^1) need only be counted and weighed at birth.

The selection of the species of the test animal to be used in the toxicant screening procedures will be determined by several considerations including cost, time, and ability to assess related human reproductive processes. The rhesus monkey or other subhuman primates, being a more comparable reproductive species, would be the animals of choice, but their cost as well as other considerations would prohibit their use in screening procedures. Laboratory rodents are economically feasible, but the relevance of the outcome of the screening to the human could be questioned. On the basis of current information, different species and strains will have to be selected for evaluating different components of the human reproductive system. Each choice would carry with it a risk of obtaining false positive and false negative data with regard to the relevance to the human female. For example, on the basis of contemporary results, the rat would be less satisfactory than the guinea pig for assessing the effects of potential toxicants on the development or the integrity of cyclic gonadotropic function.

Several neural and physiological interventions that curtail estrous cycling in the rat do not occur in the rhesus monkey and guinea pig. In addition at least some perinatal steroid manipulations that render the rat permanently anovulatory apparently do not interfere with menstrual cycles in the rhesus monkey. Thus, it is likely that many substances found to disrupt spontaneous ovulation in the rat will not do so in the human, and false positive assessments may result.

A false negative may occur if the rat is the only species used to assess the reproductive consequences of a compound. For example, the ovarian cycle of the rat does not have a spontaneous luteal phase as does the human cycle. Therefore, compounds that might interfere with the function of the corpora lutea cannot be detected in the rat. Under these circumstances another species with a comparable reproductive process, such as the guinea pig, should be considered for addition to the screening procedure.

Indexes should be calculated for mating, fecundity, female fertility, and parturition as noted below.

$$\text{mating index} = \frac{\text{number of copulations (one counted/estrous cycle)}}{\text{number of estrous cycles required}} \times 100$$

$$\text{fecundity index} = \frac{\text{number of pregnancies}}{\text{number of copulations}} \times 100$$

$$\text{fertility index} = \frac{\text{number of females conceiving}}{\text{number of females exposed}} \times 100$$

$$\text{incidence of parturition} = \frac{\text{number of parturitions}}{\text{number of pregnancies}} \times 100$$

Numbers of viable, stillborn, and cannibalized progeny are recorded for each litter, the survivors on days 1, 4, 12, and 21 postpartum noted, and litters reduced to ten pups on the fourth day of lactation for standardization. Gestational length and sex ratio are also monitored.

$$\text{live birth index} = \frac{\text{number of viable pups born}}{\text{total number of pups born}} \times 100$$

$$\text{1- or 4-day survival index} = \frac{\text{number of pups viable at location day 1 or 4}}{\text{number of pups born}}$$

$$\text{12- or 21-day survival index} = \frac{\text{number of pups viable at lactation day 12 or 21}}{\text{number of pups retained at lactation day 4}}$$

Quantitative Reproductive Toxicity Tests

Estrogen agonist–antagonist

The screening test listed previously under qualitative assessment can be used to establish dose-response relationships between estrogens and suspected estrogenic toxicants. The following discussion represents an expansion of the qualitative tests.

Neonatal exposure to various dose levels of estrogenic toxicants. These assays will result in a dose-response relationship for time of vaginal opening, ovarian degeneration and oocyte loss, and stimulation of epithelial cell height in the uterus. These end points are easy to assess, are reproducible, and are quite sensitive (μg quantities of DES, Kepone, and clomiphene are easily detected) (1–3). This is not to say that these tests have been utilized to examine a large class of compounds; however, one of the recommendations is that such compounds be studied in detail. At the present time all known estrogens are active in these assays, and hence we can expect that they will be good predictors of estrogenic potency. Likewise, such assays should identify compounds that may interfere with reproductive processes. It may be possible to extrapolate these data on relative potency to known effects of various doses of estrogens in the human, since it is well established that estrogenic responses in rodents and humans show many similarities (7–9). To this end compounds such as ethynylestradiol, DES, and estradiol should be used as standards.

Estrogen receptor analysis *in vivo* **and** *in vitro*. An extremely sensitive (picogram-nanogram range) and reproducible method for assessing relative estrogenicity involves the use of toxicants to compete with labeled estradiol in binding to uterine cytoplasmic estrogen receptors (3–6). This test involves the addition of various concentrations of the toxicant to uterine cytosol fractions in the presence of labeled estradiol. If the toxicant is estrogenic, it will compete with estradiol for binding to receptor sites, and a classical competitive inhibition curve can be obtained. From this curve a relative binding affinity (RBA) can be calculated that reflects the agonistic or antagonistic activity of the toxicant. Such estimates of potential estrogenicity may be used to extrapolate estrogenicity in humans and be of importance in approximating the relative risks in humans. Although this test is simple and requires little expense in terms of number of animals, etc., not all laboratories routinely perform such analyses. However, it is becoming more and more common and may be standard procedure in the future.

The major qualifier to such cytosol receptor assays is that certain estrogenic compounds, such as clomiphene and nafoxidine, exhibit a very low RBA and yet are more estrogenic than predicted (10). In part this is due to the slow clearance of such compounds, which provides a longer exposure time and increases the receptor occupancy *in vivo* when compared to that of more rapidly cleared estrogens. To detect such long-acting estrogens, estrogen receptors assays can be done *in vivo*. Mentioned in the section titled Qualitative Reproductive Toxicity Screen, these assays involve injecting various dose levels of the compound in immature rats and measuring the nuclear accumulation and cytoplasmic depletion of estrogen receptors. Reliable, easy to perform, and sensitive, this test requires relatively few animals. It has the disadvantage of not being a standard assay in all laboratories.

Such receptor assays can be valuable in the estimation of estrogenic potency in humans; however, the chief value of the receptor assay probably lies in its ability to detect estrogen agonist or antagonist and has the potential of elucidating primary steps in the mechanism of action of such compounds. Such insights into mechanisms may make future predictions of estrogenic toxicity a relatively simple task.

Androgen agonist–antagonist

Qualitative screening tests for androgen activity include the ventral prostate gland hypertrophy produced by administration of compounds to immature (28-day) male rats.

Additional models are necessary to evaluate androgenic effects in the following circumstances: (a) inhibition of adult female reproductive function (e.g., ovulation, behavior), and (b) masculinization of female phenotype (fetal differentiation, prepubertal development, and adulthood phenotypic transformations).

Inhibition of adult female reproductive function. The common clinical response to hyperandrogenic stimuli, is anovulation. Increasing duration of exposure or potency of the agent leads to oligomenorrhea and secondary amenorrhea. Subtle intensifications of libido are experienced by some women, particularly with more potent agents.

Laboratory testing of adult female rats requires daily evaluation of vaginal smears for no fewer than four cycles to detect interruption of the estrous cycle. A daily 1-mg dose of testosterone propionate produces diestrus within two cycles. Appropriate dose-response studies are indicated.

Masculinization of the female phenotype: fetal. After 16 days of gestation, transplacental transfer of potent androgen agonists results in a variety of imprinting and masculinizing responses that are based upon "critical periods" of organ system differentiation. Permanent alterations in the neuroendocrine regulation of the estrous cycle and male-type mating behavior are "imprinted" at lower doses of androgen than are required for disturbing reproductive tract (vaginal opening) and hepatic monooxygenase (steroid hydroxylase or dehydrogenase) activities. A 5-mg dose of testosterone propionate administered to the pregnant dam daily from day 16 to day 20 of gestation produces the masculinization response in female progeny and does not significantly disturb male differentiation. Treatment of neonatal female rats (day 1–10) with a single 1-mg dose of testosterone propionate masculinizes the hypothalamic-pituitary-ovarian axis (persistent estrus) and sexual behavior (male-type with great reliability).

Masculinization of the female phenotype: postnatal animals. Masculinization of the female phenotype and suppression of female sexual behavior and of the pubertal events is not induced permanently by treatments initiated after the postnatal period (days 1–10). Such masculinization effects produced in females tend to regress, and although vulvar changes may persist, estrous cyclicity resumes. Although these effects are clear-cut in rodents, dose extrapolation to humans is not possible.

Adulthood phenotypic transformations. Masculinization of vulva, mating behavior, and hepatic monooxygenases in adult animals are much less sensitive indicators of toxicity than the same responses in immature animals. Inhibition of ovulation in adult females is also a more sensitive indicator of toxicity than the above three parameters. Therefore, additional tests to assess phenotypic transformation in adult females are not necessary.

Hypothalamic—Pituitary Function Tests

Assay of agents that stimulate the release of gonadotropins from cells of the anterior pituitary gland

A toxicant may adversely affect reproduction by altering the rate of secretion of one or more hormones that are synthesized and released by the hypothalamus and anterior pituitary gland. Of the hormones that are secreted by the anterior pituitary gland, the gonadotropins (luteinizing hormone [LH] and follicle-stimulating hormone [FSH]) and prolactin are most closely associated with reproduction. The gonadotropins are important, because these protein hormones control ovarian function, including steroid hormone secretion, follicular development, and ovulation. Hence, if gonadotropin secretion is suppressed, ovarian function is suppressed. A toxicant could suppress the secretion of gonadotropins by acting directly on the pituitary gland or by suppressing the secretion of gonadotropin-releasing hormone (GnRH) by hypothalamic neurons.

Alternatively, a toxicant could stimulate the secretion of prolactin, and as a consequence of the hyperprolactinemia, gonadotropin secretion becomes suppressed. Prolactin secretion can be stimulated by substances that have estrogenic activity, substances that act as dopamine antagonists, substances that inhibit dopamine secretion by hypothalamic dopaminergic neurons, or substances that cause hyperplasia of prolactin-secreting cells. Some of these actions of toxicants can be assessed (e.g., by quantifying gonadotropin and prolactin secretion), whereas others cannot be evaluated in a quantitative sense (e.g., GnRH secretion). A few ways of assessing quantitatively the actions of a toxicant that may have significant effects on reproduction are listed below.

In vivo model. Since agents that stimulate the release of one gonadotropin (e.g., LH) usually affect the release of the other (viz., FSH), it is probably only necessary to measure the release of one (e.g., LH). For such studies, the estrogen-progesterone-primed female rat can be used. The Gn-releasing standard should be synthetic GnRH against which the test substance can be compared. The responsive parameter, LH in serum or plasma, can be measured by a standardized radioimmunoassay. After the ED_{50} of GnRH and the ED_{50} of the test substance have been ascertained, a standard bioassay can be performed. A three-dose assay, where each dose is replicated three to four times, may suffice. Thus, such an assay will require 18 to 24 assay animals. More animals can be used if high precision is desired. The concentration of LH in plasma or serum can be evaluated 30 to 60 minutes after the administration of the test substance and of the standard. Assuming suitable ranges of concentration and parallel slopes from the two assays and a suitable statistical analysis, such as that described by Bliss (11) for bioassays, qualitative characteristics of the assay as well as the relative potency of the unknown substance can be evaluated. If one knows the potency of GnRH in the estrogenized woman with reference to the release of LH, it is then possible to calculate the Gn-releasing activity of the test substance and express the potency in terms of GnRH.

In vitro model. The Gn-releasing properties of an unknown substance can also be measured using anterior pituitary cells maintained in monolayer culture. In this case the pituitary cells could be obtained from the rat or a suitable primate. The cells could be dispersed and established in culture. After three to five days, the test substance and GnRH can be assayed for their Gn-releasing activities, using a bioassay paradigm similar to that outlined above.

Assays of agents that inhibit the release of gonadotropins from cells of the anterior pituitary gland

The details of an *in vivo* model assay of a substance that inhibits the release of gonadotropins could be done as follows. A female rat castrated 4 to 6 weeks before testing could serve as the assay animal. (In such an animal, the concentration of LH is many times that of intact animals.) For a reference standard, 17β-estradiol could be used to suppress the release and hence concentration of LH in serum of the test animal. After the ED_{50} for estradiol and the ED_{50} for the test substance have been established, a three-dose bioassay could be conducted. After an evaluation of the parameters of the assay, it may be possible to calculate the relative potency of the test substance and express its potency in terms of 17β-estradiol.

After the potency of a test substance relative to 17β-estradiol has been established, one can then calculate the relative potency of the test substance in the human by comparing the LH-lowering effect of 17β-estradiol in castrated or postmenopausal women.

Assay of an agent that inhibits the release of prolactin from cells of the anterior pituitary gland

In vivo **model.** Although several experimental animal models could be used, the young, mature female rat would be adequate. The only pretreatment required would be a short period (3–4 days) during which the animal was handled to minimize the release of prolactin because of fright. The reference standard for the release of prolactin could be haloperidol. Prolactin release could be evaluated by measuring prolactin in the plasma or serum of the test animal. Thirty to sixty minutes after the administration of the test substance or haloperidol, serum or plasma prolactin could be measured by radioimmunoassay. After the dose-response curve (i.e., ED_{50}) is established, a bioassay could be conducted and the relative potency of the test substance calculated.

If a dose-response curve for haloperidol in women is established, one could approximate the potency of the test substance relative to haloperidol. Of course, other reference standards could be used in this prolactin release assay *in vivo*. These include thyrotropin-releasing factor and vasoactive intestinal peptide.

In vitro **model.** The ability of test substance to simulate the release of prolactin from pituitary cells could be conducted *in vitro* using pituitary cells maintained in monolayer culture. The donor could be the rat as well as a primate. After a few (3–5) days in culture, a suitable bioassay could be performed, and the potency of the test substance relative to a standard could be evaluated.

Assay of an agent that inhibits the release of prolactin from pituitary cells

In vivo **model.** An estrogen-primed female rat could be used in this assay. In such an animal the plasma concentration of prolactin is very high. For a reference standard, bromoergocriptine could be used. After dose-response curves for bromoergocriptine and for the test substance had been established, a bioassay for prolactin release inhibition could be performed, where the serum or plasma prolactin concentration is the responsive variable. After a suitable statistical analysis, one could calculate the relative potency of the test substance. As discussed above, if the dose-response relationship for bromoergocriptine in the woman (perhaps an estrogenized woman) were known, the approximate potency of the test substance relative to bromoergocriptine could be calculated.

In vitro **model.** Anterior pituitary tissue from estrogenized female rats can be used under *in vitro* conditions to test a substance for inhibition of prolactin release. Anterior pituitary tissue can be incubated in the presence of various concentrations of bromo-ergocriptine or of the test substance to establish a dose-response curve. Then, using this system, a bioassay can be conducted where the concentration of prolactin in the culture medium is the responsive variable. Pituitary cells maintained in monolayer culture could also serve as a suitable *in vitro* assay system.

Assay of the activity of an agent that alters the secretion of dopamine by hypothalamic neurons

There is no method for the quantification of the secretion by dopaminergic neurons in the human. Although there is a method for the measurement of the secretion of dopamine into hypophysial portal blood, the procedure is tedious and requires the aid of highly skilled people. Hence, this procedure is not practical as a routine procedure. Therefore, one is reduced to making turnover measurements, but such measurements are also susceptible to large error and require many animals. Thus, it is reasonable to conclude that as a routine matter, the rate of secretion of dopamine by neurons of the brain can not be done for toxicants. This is not to infer that this is not an important aspect of brain function. Indeed, it is already known that the secretory activity by dopaminergic neurons is quickly, markedly, and sometimes permanently affected by a variety of toxicants. Since dopaminergic neurons constitute an important subset of the neurons of the brain, we encourage research on this important topic.

Assay of the activity of an agent that alters the secretion of norepinephrine by hypothalamic neurons

Comments made about the secretion of dopaminergic neurons are equally applicable to neurons that secrete such biogenic agents as norepinephrine and serotonin. The available techniques for the quantitative study of neurons secreting these agents are not sufficiently advanced to enable their use in routine assays.

Assay of the activity of an agent that alters the secretion of GnRH

There is no suitable assay for such an agent at this time.

Assay of the activity of an agent that alters the secretion of hypothalamic opioid peptides

It is now clear that morphine and opiatelike peptides affect the secretion of dopamine by hypothalamic neurons and of LH by the pituitary gland. Thus, it is easy to infer an important role for the naturally occurring opiatelike peptides as well as morphine in reproduction. However, this field is too new to address in a quantitative manner or to include in a screening system. Yet it can be anticipated that at some time in the reasonable future, this shortcoming in our technical capabilities will be surmounted and these problems addressed in quantitative terms.

Blood flow of the hypothalamic-hypophysial system

Perhaps no structure in the mammal has a more complicated vasculature than the hypothalamic-hypophysial complex, consisting as it does of one component that has a high rate of perfusion and another that is avascular. Moreover, the coexistence in the pituitary stalk of portal vessels carrying blood to the anterior lobe of the pituitary from the hypothalamus and of a subependymal plexus in which pituitary hormones can pass retrograde in the stalk to the hypothalamus attests to the importance of blood flow in this area. The measurement of blood flow to the neurohypophysis (i.e., medium eminence and pars nervosa) can be measured accurately using radiolabeled microspheres. Blood flow in the anterior lobe of the pituitary can be measured using the hydrogen electrode. Thus, an area deserving of attention for effects of environmental toxicants is the hypothalamic-hypophysial complex.

Sexual behavior tests

Introduction. Alterations of mating behavior in the female rat can be used as an indicator of hypothalamic function and/or impairment of function. A voluminous literature indicates that hypothalamic neurons serve as target cells for the ovarian hormones, especially the estrogens, and that destruction of specific regions of the hypothalamus leads to abolition or disorganization of female sexual behavior (12). The studies carried out on the disturbance of sexual behavior associated with hypothalamic damage establish three points of significance to the use of the proposed sexual behavior tests: hypothalamic damage can disrupt sexual behavior without altering the neural systems that mediate pituitary-ovarian function, the disruption of sexual behavior following hypothalamic damage cannot be reversed with endocrine therapy, and the sexual disruptions show extensive phylogenetic continuity.

For these reasons, the sexual behavior system may be capable of detecting chemically induced abnormalities in hypothalamic function that cannot be detected by the other testing systems proposed. By substituting the putative toxicant for estrogen or progesterone in a standardized behavioral assay, it is possible to assess its estrogenic or progestogenic activity in hypothalamic regions other than those that modulate pituitary release of gonadotropins. Neural systems modulating female sexual behavior are by no means limited to hypothalamic structures. The tests proposed here, however, are oriented toward behavioral end points generally accepted as involving the hypothalamus. A more detailed discussion of other aspects of sexual function and the potential toxicant-induced disruption of other neural systems is available in Chapter 5.

Behavioral assay methods. Female rat sexual behavior has several components that vary in a dosage-dependent manner with estrogens and progestins. To determine whether the toxicant possesses estrogenic or progestagenic action, the experimenter would vary the dosage of the toxicant, substituting it for either estradiol benzoate (EB) or progesterone in the standard protocol of a behavior assay. The lordosis response, which includes arching of the back (13), and the number or latency of approaches that the female makes to the male (14) can be readily quantified. The testing arena should have an area of at least four square feet and contain a simple barrier or compartment. The females used in the tests should be ovariectomized and administered estrogen and progesterone (or the substituted toxicant) at times to produce mating during the dark phase of illumination. The estrogen EB (or its substitute) is administered 44 to 46 hours before the administration of progesterone (or its substitute), and the mating behavior is observed approximately four hours after administering progesterone.

A standard dose-response curve for EB would be obtained by holding the amount of progesterone constant at approximately 0.5 mg and varying the dosage of EB from 0.1 to 100 μg. When possible, the vehicle for delivering these hormones should be the same as that to be used for the toxicant and appropriate standard curves established. The progesterone standard dosage-response curve would be obtained by maintaining EB at a constant level (5–10 μg) and varying the amount of progesterone from 0.1 to 10 mg. No fewer than 10 subjects can be used to establish the behavioral response value at each dosage. Repeated mating of the same female at each dosage may be more sensitive than using different females at each dosage, but each mating should be separated by approximately 5 to 7 days.

A reliable method to determine the dose-response curve for antiestrogenic activity would be to use guinea pigs as subjects and to measure their lordosis response to the touch of the experimenter; running the index finger along the back, starting from its most caudal point. The procedure would consist of administering constant dosages of EB (5–10 μg) and, 46 hours after the initial dose of EB, a 0.5-mg dose of progesterone. When administered simultaneously with estrogen, progesterone possesses antiestrogenic properties in the guinea pig and can therefore be used as a standard to assess the antiestrogenic activity of the toxicant. Accordingly, varying dosages of the compound (0.1–10 mg) would be administered along with the EB.

The antiestrogenicity of a putative toxicant can also be evaluated in the female rat's behavior system. However, because this behavior system is relatively insensitive to the inhibitory actions or antiestrogenic actions of progesterone, an alternative antiestrogen, such as MER-25, is recommended for a comparative standard.

The toxicant can also be administered in addition to the standard doses of EB or progesterone. This can be done at the same time that estrogen and progesterone are administered to determine whether it potentiates or antagonizes the action of each of these steroids. In addition, the toxicant can be administered prior to the determination of a standard dose-response curve, and the estrogen dose-response curves can be compared with those obtained from control animals. In this way, toxicant-produced modifications of the brain areas mediating sexual behavior can be detected using a test based on a standard estrogen dose-response curve.

Relevance to humans. A positive result from these behavioral screening procedures could reflect disruption of neural, most likely hypothalamic, function and could indicate the potential for interference with human hypothalamic function. However, the manifestations of this potential hypothalamic disruption in humans will most likely be different from those in rodents.

Ovarian Toxicity

Oocyte and follicle toxicity

The ovary is responsible for two roles in reproduction: nurture and release of gametes and hormone production. Clinical and experimental data demonstrate that a variety of xenobiotic compounds can alter both aspects of ovarian function (15, 16). Multiple studies have demonstrated that one of cigarette smoking's adverse effects on the human ovary is an earlier dose-related age of menopause. The assays described here are designed to assess the effect of xenobiotics on the first aspect of ovarian function, gamete nurture. Tests for xenobiotic effects on oogenesis can be determined by including prenatal as well as postnatal treatments. Xenobiotic destruction of oocytes is of great significance because the effect is irreversible: there is no mechanism for repopulation of oocytes in the ovary.

Evidence suggests that inbred mouse strains represent the most sensitive test strains for oocyte and follicle toxicity assays (17). Additional data in other species and with other xenobiotics is needed to clarify this relationship. Inbred mouse strains also offer the advantage that they provide the logical framework for exploration of the mechanism of action as well as providing a reproducible assay system (18–20).

After treatment with the compound of interest, mice are sacrificed at varying time intervals and their ovaries removed, fixed, serially sectioned, and stained. Oocytes and follicles are quantitated using a microscope, and effect of treatment on oocyte or follicle number is determined. Follicles and oocytes are classified by the method of Zuckerman (21). This assay, although cumbersome, is easily learned and conducted by laboratory technicians.

Evidence suggests that this assay is a much more sensitive indicator of oocyte or follicle damage than alterations in fertility. Unpublished investigations at the Pregnancy Research Branch of the National Institute of Child Health and Human Development, as well as other published data, suggest that as many as 90% of all oocytes have to be destroyed before short-term alterations in fertility of the female can be observed.

The full range of specificity of the assay has yet to be determined. The assay appears to be quite sensitive and dose dependent (see Table 4 for available ED_{50}'s).

Inhibition of steroidogenesis

In developing a model system to estimate the quantitative risk of a toxicant with regard to inhibition of ovarian steroidogenesis, multiple physiological and technical aspects must be considered. These include (a) the cell-type specific sex steroids to be measured,

TABLE 4 Compounds Tested for Oocyte/Follicle Toxicity in the Murine Assay

Compound	Response	Follicle Type	ED_{50} (mg/kg)
Benzo(a)pyrene	Toxic	1-3a[a]	10
3-Hydroxybenzo(a)pyrene	Toxic	1-3a	>100
4,5-Dihydroepoxybenzo(a)pyrene	Toxic	1-3a	>100
cis-4,5-Dihydrodiolbenzo(a)pyrene	Toxic	1-3a	>100
trans-4,5-Dihydrodiolbenzo(a)pyrene	Toxic	1-3a	>100
7,8-Dihydrodiolbenzo(a)pyrene	Toxic	1-3a	<1
7,12-Dimethylbenz(a)anthracene	Toxic	1-3a	<1
3-Methylcholanthracene	Toxic	1-3a	10
Ethanol	Nontoxic		
Benzene	Nontoxic		
Toluene	Nontoxic		
Carbontetrachloride	Nontoxic		
Galactose	Toxic with prenatal exposure, nontoxic after birth	1-3a	Unknown

[a]Resting follicles as classified by Pedersen and Peters (22).

(b) the cooperative compartmental steroid biosynthesis characterizing the follicular phase, (c) the cycle-related variations in sex steroid production, (d) the key regulatory steps in steroid biosynthesis (i.e., the availability of substrate and the roles of luteinizing hormone [LH] and follicle-stimulating hormone [FSH]), (e) the available methodology, and (f) the ability to extrapolate the data between species. The focus here is placed on a model *in vitro* rather than *in vivo* because of considerations regarding the specificity of the toxic effect, the lack of interference by nervous or humoral factors present *in vivo*, the greater likelihood of intracellular interaction with the toxicant, the applicability of the test system, and the ability to extrapolate the data to human or at least primate ovarian cell types.

Estrogen, primarily 17β-estradiol progesterone, 17α-OH progesterone, androstenedione, and testosterone, are the predominant steroids produced by the human ovary during the reproductive years. Estrogen characterizes the follicular phase, with the corpus luteum producing both estrogen and progesterone and a drop in both steroids occurring at the time of menses in a nonconceptive cycle. Androgens are secreted throughout a nonconceptive cycle, with a slight rise at midcycle. Controversy still exists concerning the cell(s) of origin of follicular estrogen; both direct thecal cell secretion and granulosa cell aromatization of thecal androgen are supported in the literature (23). Because granulosa cells lack the 17,20 desmolase enzyme, the thecal and interstitial compartments are felt to be the source of C_{19} androgens. After ovulation the granulosa and thecal compartments both form the corpus luteum and produce progesterone and estrogen. Any model system using ovarian cell types *in vitro* must consider these differences as well as the overall cyclic steroid secretory pattern characteristic to the species utilized.

Regulatory steps in gonadal steroid secretion include (a) substrate (cholesterol) availability (i.e., the low-density lipoprotein fraction of plasma); (b) luteinizing-hormone (LH) induction of the 20,22-hydroxylase-desmolase steps converting cholesterol to pregnenolone, and (c) follicle-stimulating-hormone (FSH) induction of granulosa cell aromatase activity converting thecal androgens to estrogens. Since thecal steroidogenesis has not been demonstrated to depend on FSH-induced aromatization, LH stimulates thecal androgen production, and low levels of LH are required *in vivo* for adequate luteal function, some of these regulatory steps may be compartment specific.

A toxicant may not demonstrate inhibition of steroidogenesis *in vitro* and yet be active *in vivo,* if it affects selectively gonadotropin-mediated events *in vivo* or only progesterone synthesis stimulated by human chorionic gonadotropin (HCG) (24, 25), and hence be detectable only *in vivo* in a known conceptive cycle. Similarly, agents acting through prostaglandins known to induce luteal regression *in vivo* in some species (26) may be active only *in vivo,* because the agents may act not directly on the steroid-secreting cell but rather indirectly by selective ovarian veno-constrictive action. Despite these possibilities, most known inhibitors of steroidogenesis act by affecting specific enzymes in the steroid pathways (Table 5).

TABLE 5 Agents That Inhibit Steroidogenesis	
Steroidogenic Step	Inhibitor
20α hydroxylase	Amino-glutethimide phosphate
Sidechain cleavage	3-methoxybenzidine
Dehydrogenase, 3β-hydroxy-	Cyanoketone
Δ^5-steroid	Estrogens
	Azastene
	Danazol
Aromatase	4-acetoxy-androstene-3,17-dione
	4-hydroxy-androstene-3,17-dione
	1,4,6-androstatriene-3,17-dione
11β-hydroxylase	Danazol
	Metyrapone
	SKF-12185
21-hydroxylase	Danazol
17α-hydroxylase	Danazol
	SU-9055
	SU-8000
17,20 lyase	Danazol

Adequate methodology is currently available for (a) isolation of ovarian cell types (27, 28), (b) tissue or organ culture, and (c) direct radioimmunoassay of media for individual steroids without chromatography steps. If HCG stimulation of steroidogenesis is required to demonstrate an effect, serum-free media may be required, as there is some evidence that blocking factors for gonadotropins are present in serum (29); but in short-term cultures ($<$24 hours), the lack of serum factors should not present a problem for cell viability. Plating efficiency can be determined by supravital staining, and cell counts or determinations of DNA or protein can be used to normalize data. Organ cultures are more difficult to normalize because of more heterogeneous cell populations, less well-defined culture conditions, and more difficult assessments of cell viability, but tissue wet weights can be used. Enzymatic dispersion techniques are available (25), but they add considerable time to the procedure and do not solve the problem of cell heterogenicity. Furthermore, if gonadotropin stimulation is required, highly purified enzyme preparations (i.e., collagenase) are necessary to avoid protese contamination and alterations in membrane-bound protein receptors (30). Hence, because of ease of culture, purity of cell type, and active basal steroidogenesis, isolated granulosa cell cultures, with or without added C_{19} androgen substrate, represent attractive models for evaluation of a potential toxicant's effect on steroidogenesis (Table 6).

Cell-cell interactions may control the pattern of ovarian steroidogenesis as evidenced by the so-called "spontaneous luteinization" that granulosa cells undergo when placed in tissue culture independent of when they are harvested in the follicular phase (31). The removal of the cells from their approximation to the thecal layer, contact with follicular fluid, or disruption of intimate cell-to-cell contact appears to alter their steroidogenic potential and morphologic appearance *in vitro*. For these reasons the use of intact follicle walls without separation of the thecal and granulosa compartments may have to be considered as a test system if problems are encountered with isolated cell systems.

Selection of the species for use depends primarily on availability of adequate numbers of physiologically matured follicles or corpora lutea. While diethylstilbestrol-treated immature rats can be used as a source of ovarian cells (32), the numbers of cells are small and require a substantial time investment for collection. Domestic animals, by contrast, have much larger follicles, and the use of slaughterhouse material of a polyovulatory species minimizes the precollection time investment. Pigs and cows are the most desirable large animals to use in this regard, and both have an extensive literature available regarding their reproductive cycles, cell collection techniques, and tissue culture. The cell system chosen should be an easily exploitable model system in which known inhibitors of steroidogenesis in both human and animal systems can be studied *in vitro* to validate the animal model and the data extrapolated to humans for more general application to quantitative risk assessment of other suspicious compounds.

TABLE 6 Features of Ovarian Cell Preparations, *In Vitro*, Potentially Useful in Xenobiotic Inhibition of Steroidogenesis[a]

Characteristic	Separated		Intact Follicle Walls (Thecal and Granulosa)	Luteal Cells	Stromal or Interstitial Cells
	Granulosa Cells	Thecal Cells			
Predominant steroids secreted (in order of amount)	Progesterone Estrogens[c] (only with added substrates)	Androgens[b] Estrogens Progesterone	Estrogen Androgens[b] Progesterone	Progesterone Estrogen	Androgens[b]
Steroid production independent of cycle stage	−	−	−	−	+
Steroid production not dependent on another cell type	−	+	−	+	+
Active basal steroidogenesis	+	+	+	+	−
Purity	+	−	NA	+	+
Ease of isolation	+	−	−	+[d]	+[d]

[a]A plus (+) indicates presence and a minus (−), absence of a characteristic listed in first column. NA means not applicable.
[b]Testosterone and androstenedione in varying proportion.
[c]Estradiol-17β and estrone in varying proportion.
[d]Dispersed cell culture requires enzymatic digestion; organ culture requires only excision.

REFERENCES

1. Gellert, R. J., Bakke, J. L. and Lawrence, N. L.: Persistent estrus and altered estogen sensitivity in rats treated neonatally with clomiphene citrate. Fertil. Steril. 22: 224–250, 1971.

2. Clark, J. H. and McCormack, S. A.: The effect of clomid and other triphenylethylene derivatives during pregnancy and the neonatal period. J. Steroid Biochem. 12: 47, 1980.

3. Eroschenko, V. and Palmiter, R.: Estrogenicity of kepone in birds and mammals. In: Estrogens in the Environment, J. McLachlan, Ed., Elsevier/North Holland: New York; pp. 305–326, 1980.

4. Clark, J. H. and Peck, E. J., Jr.: Female Sex Steroids: Receptors and Function: Springer-Verlag: Berlin; 245 pp., 1979.

5. Katzenellenbogen, J., Katzenellenbogen, B., Tatee, T., Robertson, D. and Landratter, S.: The chemistry of estrogens and antiestrogens. In: Estrogens in the Environment, J. McLachlan, Ed., Elsevier/North Holland: New York; pp. 33, 1980.

6. Kupfer, D. and Bulger, W.: Estrogenic properties of DDT and its analogs. In: Estrogens in the Environment, J. McLachlan, Ed., Elsevier/North Holland: New York; pp. 239–263, 1980.

7. Chan, L. and O'Malley, B. W.: Mechanism of action of sex steroid-hormones. I. N. Engl. J. Med. 294: 1322–1328, 1976.

8. Chan, L. and O'Malley, B. W.: Mechanism of action of sex steroid-hormones. II. N. Engl. J. Med. 294: 1372–1381, 1976.

9. Chan, L. and O'Malley, B. W.: Mechanism of action of sex steroid-hormones. III. N. Engl. J. Med. 294: 1430–1437, 1976.

10. Clark, J. H., Anderson, J. N. and Peck, E. J., Jr.: Estrogen receptor antiestrogen complex: atypical binding by uterine nuclei and effects on uterine growth. Steroids 22: 707–713, 1973.

11. Bliss, C. I.: Statistical methods in vitamin research. In: Vitamin Methods, P. György, Ed., Academic Press: New York; pp. 448–609, 1951.

12. Pfaff, D. W.: Estrogens and Brain Function: Neural Analysis of a Hormone-Controlled Mammalian Reproductive Behavior. Springer-Verlag: New York; 272 pp., 1980.

13. Gerall, A. A. and McCrady, R. E.: Receptivity scores of female rats stimulated either manually or by males. J. Endrocrinol. 46: 55–59, 1970.

14. McClintock, M. K. and Adler, N. T.: The role of the female during copulation in the wild and domestic Norway rat. Behavior 67(1–2): 67–96, 1978.

15. Mattison, D. R.: How xenobiotic compounds can destroy oocytes. Contemp. Ob. Gyn. 15: 157–169, 1980.

16. Mattison, D. R. and Thorgeirsson, S. S.: Smoking and industrial pollution and their effects on menopause and ovarian cancer. Lancet 1: 187–188, 1978.

17. Mattison, D. R.: Difference in sensitivity of rat and mouse primoridal oocytes to destruction by polycyclic aromatic hydrocarbons. Chem. Biol. Interact. 28: 133–137, 1979.

18. Mattison, D. R. and Thorgeirsson, S. S.: Gonadal arylhydrocarbon hydroxylase in rats and mice. Cancer Res. 38: 1368–1373, 1978.

19. Mattison, D. R. and Thorgeirsson, S. S.: Ovarian arylhydrocarbon hydroxylase activity and primordial occyte toxicity of polycyclic aromatic hydrocarbons in mice. Cancer Res. 39: 3471–3475, 1979.

20. Mattison, D. R., West, D. M. and Menard, R. A.: Differences in benzo(*a*)pyrene metabolic profile in rat and mouse ovary. Biochem. Pharmacol. 25: 2101–2104, 1979.

21. Zuckerman, S.: The Ovary. Academic Press: New York; 600 pp., 1962.

22. Pedersen, T. and Peters, H.: Proposal for a classification of oocytes and follicles in the mouse ovary. J. Reprod. Fertil. 17: 555–557, 1968.

23. Armstrong, D. T. and Dorrington, J. H.: Estrogen biosynthesis in the ovaries and testes. In: Regulatory Mechanisms Affecting Gonadal Hormone Action, Advances in Sex Hormone Research, J. A. Thomas, and R. L. Singhal, Eds., University Park Press: Baltimore; 3: 217–258, 1977.

24. Stouffer, R. L., Nixon, W. E. and Hodgen, G. E.: Estrogen inhibition of basal and gonadotropin-stimulated progesterone production by Rhesus monkey luteal cells *in vitro*. Endocrinol. 101: 1157–1163, 1977.

25. Williams, M. T., Roth, M. S., Marsh, J. M. and LeMaire, W. J.: Inhibition of Human chorionic gonadotropin-induced progesterone synthesis by estradiol in isolated human luteal cells. J. Clin. Endocrinol. Metab. 48: 437–440, 1979.

26. Goldberg, V. J. and Ramwell, P. W.: Role of prostaglandins in reproduction. Physiol. Rev. 55: 325–351, 1975.

27. McNatty, K. P., Makris, A., DeGrazia, C., Osathanondh, R. and Ryan, K. J.: The production of progesterone, androgens and estrogens by granulosa-cells, thecal tissue, and stromal tissue from human ovaries, *in vitro*. J. Clin. Endocrinol. Metab. 49: 687–699, 1979.

28. Haney, A. F. and Schomberg, D. W.: Steroidal modulation of progesterone secretion by granulosa-cells from large porcine follicles: a role for androgens and estrogens in controlling steroidogenesis. Biol. Reprod. 19: 242, 1978.

29. Erickson, G. F., Wang, C. and Hsueh, A. J. W.: FSH induction of functional LH receptors in granulosa cells cultured in a chemically defined medium. Nature 279: 336–338, 1979.

30. Gulyas, B. J., Yuan, L. C. and Hodgen, G. D.: Progesterone production by dispersed monkey (*Macaca Mulatta*) luteal cells after exposure to trypsin. Steroids 35: 43–51, 1980.

31. Channing, C. P.: Influences of the *in vivo* and *in vitro* hormonal environment upon luteinization of granulosa cells in tissue culture. Recent Prog. Horm. Res. 26: 589–622, 1970.

32. Hall, P. F. and Young, D. G.: Site of action of trophic hormones upon the biosynthetic pathways to steroid hormones. Endocrinol. 82: 559, 1968.

II. GLOSSARY OF TERMS USED IN FEMALE REPRODUCTION

adenosis—a nonneoplastic glandular disease that occurs in the uterine arnix and upper vagina.

amenorrhea—absence or abnormal cessation of the menses.

androgen—a class of steroid hormones produced in the gonads and adrenal cortex that regulate masculine sexual characteristics; a generic term for agents that encourage the development of or prevent changes in male sex characteristics; a precursor of estrogens.

androgen antagonist or **antiandrogen**—agent that opposes or impedes the action of an androgen.

anovulation—suspension or cessation of the escape of ova from the follicles.

corpus luteum—an endocrine body formed in ovary at site of ruptured Graafian follicle that secretes an estrogenic and progestagenic hormone.

diestrus—quiescent period following ovulation in the estrous cycle of female mammals in which the uterus prepares for reception of a fertilized ovum.

dopamine or **hydroxytyramine**—an intermediate in tyrosine catabolism and the precursor of norepinephrine and epinephrine.

ectopic pregnancy—pregnancy occurring outside the uterine cavity
egg—female sexual cell.

estradiol—an estrogenic hormone ($C_{18}H_{24}O_2$) produced by follicle cells of the vertebrate ovary; provokes estrus and proliferation of the human endometrium.

estrogen—estrogenic hormone; generic term for various natural or synthetic substances that produce estrus.

estrogen agonist—an agent that has a biological activity similar to that of the physiological estrogens.

estrogen antagonist or **antiestrogen**—agent that opposes or impedes the action of an estrogen.

estrus—phase of the sexual cycle of female mammals characterized by willingness to mate and in intact animals when ovulation occurs.

follicle (ovarian)—one of the vascular bodies in the ovary, containing the oocytes.

follicle-stimulating hormone or **FSH**—a glycoprotein hormone secreted by the anterior pituitary of vertebrates that promotes spermatogenesis and stimulates growth and secretion of the Graafian follicle.

galactorrhea—continued discharge of milk from the breasts in the intervals between nursing or after weaning.

gonadotropin—a substance that acts to stimulate the gonads.

Graafian follicle—mature mammalian ovum with its surrounding epithelial cells.

gynecomastia—excessive development of the male mammary glands, sometimes leading to milk secretion.

hypothalamic-pituitary-ovarian axis—the hormonal interactions that link and control female reproduction.

hypothalamic-hypophyseal complex—the structural and hormonal relationships between the hypothalamus and the pituitary.

lactation—the production of milk; the period following childbirth during which milk is formed in the breasts.

luteinizing hormone or **LH**—glycoprotein hormone secreted by the adenohypophysis of vertebrates that stimulates hormone production by interstitial cells of gonads.

menopause—natural physiologic cessation of menustration, normally occurring in the last half of the fourth decade.

oligomenorrhea—prolongation of menstrual cycle beyond average limits.

oocyte—female ovarian germ cell present after birth.

ovarian cyclicity—the periodic changes observed in the ovary associated with follicular growth, ovulation, and corpus luteum function.

ovulation—discharge of an ovum or ovule from a Graafian folicle in the ovary.

parturition—labor; giving birth.

postpartum estrus—estrus with ovulation and corpus luteum production which occurs in some species immediately after birth of offspring.

progesterone—a steroid hormone ($C_{21}H_{30}O_2$) produced in corpus luteum, placenta, testes, and adrenals that plays a physiological role in the luteal phase of menstrual cycle and maintenance of pregnancy; also an intermediate in biosynthesis of androgens and estrogens.

prolactin—a protein hormone produced by adenohypophysis that stimulates secretion of milk and promotes functional activity of the corpus luteum.

prostaglandins—various 20-carbon-atom compounds, formed from essential fatty acids, that physiologically affect the female reproductive organs, the nervous system, and metabolism.

puberty—period at which the generative organs become capable of reproduction.

relative binding affinity—the degree to which a ligand, compared to standard ligand, is bound to a receptor.

secondary amenorrhea—any case in which the menses appeared at puberty but have been suppressed.

steroidogenesis—enzymatic steps converting acetate and cholesterol to sex steroids, glucosteroids, or mineralocorticoids.

testosterone—a biologically potent androgenic steroid which may be released from the gonads and adrenal glands.

virilization or **masculinization**—the assumption of male characteristics by a female because of excessive production of androgenic substances or masculinizing tumors of the ovaries.

CHAPTER 3
CONSIDERATIONS IN EVALUATING RISK TO MALE REPRODUCTION

J. Michael Bedford
Cornell Medical School
New York, NY 10021

INTRODUCTION

During evolution the reproductive patterns of mammals, including man, were determined to a considerable extent by the nature of the environment. Similarly today a variety of natural environmental factors may alter reproductive activity and fertility. Potential hazards to man's reproductive state are present in the environment as pollutants whose effects are often not likely to be clear-cut. Thus, sensitive assessment systems are needed. However, it is not clear how the potential effects on male reproduction can best be assessed.

Detailed information about many aspects of male reproduction exists, but there is little firsthand experience with detection in animals of subtle effects of either new chemicals or environmental hazards. The task of detecting effects that may be reflected only marginally in fertility performance is made more difficult by the variability of different reproductive parameters such as the concentration of sperm in an ejaculate, the total number of sperm ejaculated, and the sperm morphology within a population of "normal" men in our society. Hence, our understanding of the reasons for this variation and our ability to evaluate subtle responses to environmental hazards is minimal, and it is important to recognize the embryonic state of our abilities in this regard.

It is clear that changes in human reproductive function induced by environmental hazards might be reflected in reproductive behavior; in circulating levels of hormones such as follicle-stimulating hormone (FSH), luteinizing hormone (LH), and testosterone; or in testicular and epididymal function as evidenced by spermatogenic activity, fertilizing potential of the ejaculate, and ability of the sperm genome to support normal development after fertilization. Monitoring of a human population for the normality of any of these functions and assessment of the risk of certain levels of a chemical hazard require objective criteria that are measurable in man and, when a new chemical is to be evaluated, in an appropriate animal model. Ejaculates of human and of animal semen contain a considerable heterogeneity of spermatozoa, and several parameters of ejaculates may vary considerably from sample to sample. Nonetheless, there is now a reasonable knowledge of many facets of the normal physiology and of the variations to be expected for many specific parameters in animal models and to a lesser extent for man. The guidelines described below are based on current knowledge of the physiology of male reproduction in mammals, including man, and suggest an approach to risk assessment of existing and potential chemical hazards for reproductive function.

Aspects of the Problem

The single most sensitive and important parameter for human fertility is the total number of motile sperm in an ejaculate (1, 2). It has not been possible to set an exact limit on the minimal number of motile sperm per ejaculate, or what is more commonly reported as concentration of sperm or semen, necessary for fertility in man. A male ejaculating as few as 1×10^6 sperm per milliliter may prove fertile occasionally (3), but in most cases low numbers of sperm per ejaculate bear an obvious relationship to infertility. For example, sperm concentrations below 10 million, of from 10 to 20 million, and from 20 to 40 million per milliliter are associated with a risk of infertility that is, respectively, tenfold, fivefold, and threefold higher than for individuals with normal spermatozoal concentration, that is, 60 to 160 million per milliliter (4). Because another study (5) shows that relative risks are fourfold and twofold higher for men with sperm concentrations of below 10 million and between 10 and 20 million per milliliter, respectively, it is quite possible that a twofold reduction in sperm concentration in individuals with sperm counts below 40 million per milliliter will double the incidence of infertility. Several characteristics of human semen and testicular function reflect a low efficiency (2, 6). Human testes may function often at the threshold of pathology (2, 7, 8) and may be particularly sensitive to toxic agents compared with the testes of animals commonly used to study testicular function.

The yield of spermatozoa from spermatogonia, the rate of sperm production per gram of testis, and the percentage of morphologically normal sperm in ejaculates are lowest in man among the many mammals studied (2, 6–8). The median number of sperm ($\sim$200 $\times$ 10^6 per ejaculate) is only fourfold higher than the value (50 $\times$ 10^6 per ejaculate) below which fertility becomes significantly reduced (9). In contrast, the number of sperm in an ejaculate of bull semen (7 $\times$ 10^9), is 1400-fold higher than the value of 5 $\times$ 10^6 sufficient to achieve maximal fertility by artificial insemination (10), and a smaller animal, the rabbit, also shows a large differential. It is possible that a given set of conditions in the environment may cause infertility in man more readily than in experimental animals. Several agents, including radiation (11–14), chemotherapeutic drugs (15–18), and dibromochloropropane (19–22), reduce motile sperm concentrations and affect fertility.

Selection of an Animal Model

Evaluation of compounds for potential risk to human males requires one or more animal models. The selection and use of these models for testing end points that signify a reproductive hazard generally is more specialized than that for most toxicology or mutagenesis testing. The relevant end points depend on integrated functional aspects that can be monitored with ease only in certain species. The use of two species reduces the possibility of missing a hazardous agent during testing.

Parallel testing of both rat and rabbit seems most suitable. Although a number of laboratory or domesticated species might be used, rabbits and rats offer several advantages in comparison to dogs and subhuman primates. Rabbits have a high, predictable libido that may be useful in assessing risks to sexual behavior. More importantly, all sequential phases of the conception process (i.e., endocrine function, spermatogenesis, sperm maturation, ejaculation, sperm capacitation in the female, and fertilization) are easily evaluated, quantified, and manipulated throughout the year. The ability to characterize the whole ejaculate quantitatively and qualitatively and the ability to collect the ejaculate with ease using an artificial vagina make the rabbit a key test model for sensitive assessment of possible harmful effects of environmental agents on male reproduction.

The rat is also a very useful model and is preferable to the mouse or hamster because of the rat's widespread use in toxicological research, the large base of knowledge of its reproductive processes, its relatively low cost, its convenient size for weighing organs, and the fact that it breeds readily under laboratory conditions. The rat is less useful than the rabbit, because more of the measurements require invasive procedures and/or sacrifice of the individual. The characteristics of several potential models are summarized in Table 7 (1, 23).

TABLE 7   Criteria for Evaluation of Male Reproduction in Favored Animal Models and Man

	Mouse	Rat	Rabbit (New Zealand White)	Dog (beagle)	Monkey (rhesus)	Man
Duration of cycle of seminiferous epithelium (days)	8.6	12.9	10.7	13.6	9.5	16.0
Life span of						
B-type spermatogonia (days)	1.5	2.0	1.3	4.0	2.9	6.3
L+Z[a] spermatocytes (days)	4.7	7.8	7.3	5.2	6.0	9.2
P+D[a] spermatocytes (days)	8.3	12.2	10.7	13.5	9.5	15.6
Golgi spermatids (days)	1.7	2.9	2.1	6.9	1.8	7.9
Cap spermatids (days)	3.5	5.0	5.2	3.0	3.7	1.6
Fraction of lifespan as						
B-type spermatogonia	0.11	0.10	0.08	0.19	0.19	0.25
Primary spermatocyte	1.00	1.00	1.00	1.00	1.00	1.00
Round spermatid	0.41	0.40	0.43	0.48	0.35	0.38
Testes wt (g)	0.2	3.7	6.4	12.0	49	34
Daily sperm production						
Per gram testis (10^6/g)	28	24	25	20	23	4.4
Per male (10^6)	5	86	160	300	1100	125
Sperm reserves in cauda (at sexual rest; 10^6)	49	440	1600	?[b]	5700	420
Transit time (days) through (at sexual rest)						
Caput + Corpus epididymides	3.1	3.0	3.0	?	4.9	1.8
Cauda epididymides	5.6	5.1	9.7	?	5.6	3.7

TABLE 7 (Continued)

	Mouse	Rat	Rabbit (New Zealand White)	Dog (beagle)	Monkey (rhesus)	Man
Evaluation possible of						
Testis size in situ	No	Yes	Yes	Yes	Yes	Yes
Number of testis spermatids	Yes	Yes	Yes	Yes	Yes	Yes
Testis histology	Yes	Yes	Yes	Yes	Yes	Yes
Quantitatively collected semen	No	No	Yes	Yes	Yes[c]	Yes
Feasible fertility tests						
Natural mating	Yes	Yes	Yes	No	No	No
Artificial insemination	No	No	Yes	No	No	No
In vitro	Yes	Yes	Yes	Yes	Yes	Yes
Analysis of seminal plasma for agent	No	No	Yes	Yes	Yes[c]	Yes
Sufficient sperm for in vitro testing	No	No	Yes	Yes	Yes	Yes
Sufficient blood to assay 3 hormones	Yes	Yes	Yes	Yes	Yes	Yes
Longitudinal hormonal analyses	No	Yes	Yes	Yes	Yes	Yes

[a]L = leptotene, Z = zygotene, P = pachytene, D = diplotene.
[b]A question mark indicates unclear or inadequate data.
[c]Semen obtained by electroejaculation.
Source: Adapted from Refs. 1 and 23.

Tests for Evaluating Reproductive Damage

We reviewed a wide spectrum of test systems. Table 8 (24–56) lists tests that were considered to be suitable for qualitative and quantitative risk assessment (for detailed consideration, see the Appendix to this chapter). Table 9 (including Refs. 57–70) lists additional tests that were considered but rejected because they are insensitive, redundant, not cost effective, too difficult to perform unless within a research setting, not validated, too controversial, or in need of further development.

The tests in Table 8 evaluate the endocrine control of male reproduction and the number and quality of sperm produced, or they measure fertility. Since fertility is related to the number of normal spermatozoa in the ejaculate, the analyses of seminal quality are indirect measures of fertility. However, comprehensive seminal analysis is a much more sensitive end point for detection of a toxic effect than a breeding experiment using natural mating, because in experimental animals the number of sperm ejaculated greatly exceeds the number necessary for fertility (10, 71). The various tests are stratified into a sequence (tests 1–3, S, E) ranging from a preliminary screen to more detailed studies.

Coefficients of variation (CV) might be used to determine the sensitivity of a study that compares treated animals with controls (see Appendix). Generally, measurements of testicular and epididymal sperm numbers give highly reproducible values in control animals with coefficients of variation between animals of 15% or less (24). This degree of reproducibility ensures that the test will be quite sensitive, even with relatively few animals (Table 10). Although there is appreciable variation (CV $\cong$ 70%) in sperm concentration or total number of sperm per ejaculate in semen collected from rabbits or bulls (72, 73), this variation can be reduced somewhat by using a uniform interval between seminal collections and standardized procedures in chronic studies. Sperm motility and morphology are much more constant than sperm number or concentration, especially within individuals of a species (10, 74). These two assays usually are performed in a subjective manner, and efforts must be made to minimize this subjectivity (2). In some species motility can be evaluated objectively by measurements made on time exposure negatives (75) or probably better on videotape recordings (49). Morphology of spermatozoa from individuals always should be compared to control samples analyzed concurrently by the same observer. The slides and/or videotapes should be retained for validation by an outside observer.

TABLE 8 Tests Considered Useful for Screening Toxic Compounds[a]

Test	Rat	Rabbit	Human	Reference
Body Weight	1–3	1–3	S, E	
Testis				
Size in situ	1–3	1–3	S, E	24–26
Weight	1–3	1–3	NP	24–27
Spermatid reserves	1–3[b]	1–3[b]	NP	24, 25, 27–30
Gross histology	1–3[c]	1–3[c]	NP	26, 31–34
Nonfunctional tubules (%)	2,3[b]	2,3[b]	NP	13, 18, 35
Tubules with lumen sperm (%)	2,3	2,3	NP	26, 32, 33
Tubule diameter	2,3	2,3	NP	26
Counts of leptotene spermatocytes	1–3	1–3	NP	32, 34
Epididymis				
Weight of distal half	1–3	1–3	NP	25, 27
Number of sperm in distal half	1–3	1–3	NP	27, 36, 37
Motility of sperm, distal end (%)	1–3	1–3	NP	38–40
Gross sperm morphology, distal end (%)	1	1	NP	41, 42
Detailed sperm morphology, distal end (%)	2,3	2,3	NP	6, 41, 42
Gross histology	NA	NA	NP	
Accessory Sex Glands				
Weight of vesicular glands	1–3	NA	NP	26, 27, 43
Weight of total accessory sex glands	NA	1–3	NP	26, 27, 43
Semen				
Total volume	NP	1–3	E	2, 24, 26, 44–46
Gel-free volume	NP	1–3	NA	24, 26, 44–46
Sperm concentration	NP	1–3	E	2, 24, 26, 44–46
Total sperm/ejaculate	NP	1–3	E	24, 26, 44–48
Total sperm/day of abstinence	NP	1–3	E	2, 24, 26, 48
Sperm motility, visual (%)	NP	1–3	E	2, 26
Sperm motility, videotape (% and velocity)	NP	2,3	E	2, 49
Gross sperm morphology	NP	1	NA	2
Detailed sperm morphology	NP	2,3	E	2, 42, 50
Concentration of agent in sperm	NP	NA	NA	
Concentration of agent in seminal plasma	NP	3[d]	E[d]	
Concentration of agent in blood	NP	3[d]	E[d]	
Biochemical analyses of sperm/seminal plasma	NP	NA	NA	2, 46, 51
Endocrine				
Luteinizing hormone	2,3	2,3	E	52, 53
Follicle-stimulating hormone	2,3	2,3	S, E	52, 53
Testosterone	2,3	2,3	E	52, 53
Gonadotropin-releasing hormone	2,3	2,3	E	52, 53
Fertility				
Ratio exposed: pregnant females	1–3	1–3	NP	54
Number embryos or young per pregnant female	1–3	1–3	NP	54
Ratio viable embryos: corpora lutea	1–3	NA	NP	54
Ratio implantation: corpora lutea	1–3	NA	NP	54
Number 2–8 cell eggs	3[b]	NA	NP	55
Number unfertilized eggs	3[e]	NA	NP	55
Number abnormal eggs	3[e]	NA	NP	55
Sperm per ovum	3[e]	NA	NP	55
Number of corpora lutea	3[e]	NA	NP	
In Vitro				
Incubation of sperm in agent	NA	3[f]	E[f]	
Hamster egg penetration test	NA	NA	E	56

TABLE 8 (Continued)

[a]Test 1 = initial at maximum tolerated dose (MTD), or MTD and 0.7 MTD, run for exactly six cycles of the seminiferous epithelium. A similarly significant change (probably >15%) in any criterion would be evidence of an effect.

Test 2 = dose response at MTD, at −1 and −2 log dose, and down to human level if known or until no response is obtained in any test; run for exactly six cycles of the seminiferous epithelium.

Test 3 = long term, reversibility; several doses and time periods. Expose to at least three doses for at least 6 cycles of the seminiferous epithelium (kill 1/3 of males) and then allow recovery for 6 cycles (kill 1/3 of males) and 12 cycles (kill 1/3 of males). Recovery at 12 cycles after termination of treatment should be to at least 90% of control level to show complete reversibility.

S = procedure useful for screening humans in industrial setting.

E = procedure useful for studying individuals thought to be exposed to an agent. Evaluation of human semen should use samples obtained after 2 to 5 days of abstinence with samples taken over time.

NA = not necessary.

NP = not practical or possible.

[b]Especially important when studying recovery.

[c]Save tissue from level 1 test, fix in Bouins, for possible later use.

[d]In 3 samples taken near end of treatment and then in additional samples to get clearance rate.

[e]Female rats killed 18–24 hours after mating to evaluate fertility, sperm penetrating ability, and sperm transport.

[f]If compound is detected in seminal plasma of rabbit or man, incubate both rabbit sperm and human sperm from normal donors and determine a dose response of sperm to the drug *in vitro*. Evaluate percentage of motile sperm over time at 37° or *in vitro* penetration of hamster oocyte.

All of the tests listed in Table 8 are feasible in most well-equipped laboratories. The phase-contrast microscope and video micrography equipment (estimated additional cost: $6000) are the only nonstandard requirements. The training period necessary to conduct the tests in an accurate and precise manner is not excessive.

The tests selected can be used to (a) detect an effect of a test compound on male reproduction and (b) serve as a basis for estimating an acceptable level of exposure.

The tests listed will yield quantitative data that are amenable to efficient statistical analyses and that have a sufficient range of values to enable establishment of dose-response curves. The variability of the tests is shown in Table 10 for most parameters.

The proposed tests are for the most part quite specific for reproductive toxicity. Results of each test should not be affected by other body systems or, except for a possible decrease in testosterone level, cause changes in other aspects of body function.

Any subchronic or chronic test used to evaluate effects of an agent on male reproduction must extend over 6 cycles of the seminiferous epithelium, when it is assumed that an agent bioaccumulates to a steady state within 1 cycle (23). This interval is based on (a) the time needed to reach a steady state concentration of

TABLE 9   Reasons for Rejection of Potential Evaluation Tests
Considered by Male Reproductive Subgroup

Test	References	Reasons for rejection[a]
Tonometric measurement of testicular consistency	26, 57	US (rat), NV (rabbit), FR (human)
Qualitative testicular histology	24, 31, 34	I
Stage of cycle at which spermiation occurs	24, 31, 34	RR, UR
Quantitative testicular histology		
Counts of degenerating germ cells	18, 35, 58	UR
Complete germ cell counts	18, 35, 58	UR, $$
Stem cell counts	18, 35, 58	UR, $$, FR (rabbit)
Relative frequency of stages of cycle	18, 35, 58	UR, I
Epididymal histology	59, 60	I, NR
Biochemistry of epididymal fluids	2, 61	NR
Histology of accessory sex glands	62	NR
Biochemical analysis of sperm	2	NR, $$
Sperm membrane characteristics	63, 64	NV, FR
Biochemical analysis of seminal plasma	65	NR
Evaluation of sperm metabolism	65, 66	NR, $$
Fluorescent Y bodies in spermatozoa	67, 68	NV, NR
Flow cytometry of spermatozoa	69	UR, NV, FR
Karyotyping human sperm pronuclei	70	FR
Cervical mucous penetration test		UR (human)
Studies on prepuberal animals		NR (rat, rabbit)[b]

[a]US = unsuitable for species
NV = not validated
RR - redundant
I = insensitive
NR = not relevant
UR = only in specialist lab
FR = future research
$$ = too costly

[b]Studies on animals treated prior to puberty have not been included for the following reasons. It would involve a redetermination of maximum-tolerated-dose levels for young, growing animals. The choice of age period of exposure is a complex topic and sufficient time was not available to adequately consider this. Humans are exposed to many of the agents that would cause reproductive problems primarily through occupational exposure after puberty. Some agents (radiation, cyclophosphamide) that cause reproductive problems with prepuberal exposure also affect postpuberal males. Nonetheless, unique developmental processes occur in testicular development prior to and during puberty, and therefore a possibility exists that some agents would only affect the prepuberal male. The group of tests proposed in Table 8 would provide a sensitive measure of such effects, if animals exposed at any time during puberty or throughout their development were analyzed after reaching sexual maturity.

agent in the target organs of the rabbit or rat, (b) the concepts that an agent acting directly or indirectly on the germinal epithelium may act on a specific type of cell and that affected germ cells may develop for some time before they degenerate, (c) the fact that damage to germ cells is most evident by absence of certain *types* of germ cells, and (d) qualitative change in germ cells may not be readily discernible until active spermatozoa pass into the cauda epididymidis or ejaculated semen. The present protocol assumes that attainment of a steady state concentration of an agent requires an interval equal to one cycle of the seminiferous epithelium. Formation of primary spermatocytes from renewing spermatogonia in the

TABLE 10   Approximate Variation Between Animals for Suggested Test Criteria (CV)[a] Coefficient of Variation (%)

Criterion	Rat model[b] (Wistar)	Rabbit model[c] (New Zealand White)	Rabbit model[c] (Dutch Belted)
Body weight	20	37	9.5
Testis			
Weight	5	18	20
Size in situ	NA[a]	9	20
Spermatid reserves per testis	11	24	28
Spermatid reserves per gram	8	9	
Tubule diameter	–[e]	5	11
Epididymis			
Weight of distal half	13	13	20
Number of sperm in distal half	20	52	30
Motility of sperm, distal end (%)	–	–	12
Gross sperm morphology, distal end (%)	–	–	
Detailed sperm morphology, distal end (%)	–	–	8
Accessory sex glands			
Weight vesicular glands	26	100[f]	100[f]
Weight total accessory sex glands		25	
Semen			
Total volume	NA	–	50
Gel-free volume	NA	40	50
Sperm concentration	NA	41	60
Total sperm per ejaculate	NA	–	75
Total sperm per day of abstinence	NA	28	–
Sperm motility, visual (%)	NA	–	12
Sperm motility, videotape (%)	NA	–	–
Gross sperm morphology	NA	–	–
Detailed sperm morphology	NA	–	–
Concentration of agent in seminal plasma	NA	–	8
Concentration of agent in blood	NA	–	–
Endocrine			
Luteinizing hormone	80		
Follicle-stimulating hormone	65		
Testosterone	33		
Gonadotrophin-releasing-hormone stimulation	–		
Fertility[f]			
Ratio of exposed to pregnant females			15
No. embryos or young per exposed female			20%
No. embryos or young per pregnant female			15%
Ratio of embryos to corpora lutea			10%

[a]Data are not available to allow calculation of sensitivity of the tests used with humans.
[b]Ref. 27.
[c]Refs. 25, 37, and 44.
[d]NA = not applicable.
[e]– = data not available.
[f]For controls: with treatment, variability may be greater.

rat requires about 1.5 cycles, and spermiation occurs about 3 cycles of the seminiferous epithelium after those sperm have become primary spermatocytes. Passage of sperm through the epididymis into the distal cauda or ejaculated semen requires 1.0 to 1.5 cycles, depending on the species and frequency of ejaculation. Consequently, if an agent acted on A-type spermatogonia, a decrease in number of sperm ejaculated or in the fertility of sperm from the cauda epididymidis might not occur for 5 to 6 cycles (1.5 + 3.0 + 1.0 = 5.5 cycles) of the seminiferous epithelium. If the agent resulted in degeneration of pachytene spermatocytes, an alteration in semen characteristics or fertility might be expected to occur after 4.0 to 4.5 cycles. However, with continuous exposure to the test compound, such a lesion would remain detectable in the semen or by examination of testicular histology at the end of 6 cycles of the seminiferous epithelium.

By testing male rats or rabbits for their fertility after 5 cycles, a depression in fertility caused by a compound inducing a qualitative change in sperm function should be detectable, since this probably would affect spermatocytes or spermatids. Allowing 6 to 8 days of sexual rest between the end of fertility testing and necropsy of test males after 6 cycles provides time for restoration of the normal population of sperm in the cauda epididymidis in males receiving doses that do not suppress daily sperm production. If sperm production is low in test males, the reserve level in the cauda will reflect this, but sufficient sperm may still be present to allow assessment of sperm motility and morphology.

For these reasons, evaluation of an agent, administered chronically, for effects on male reproduction should include fertility tests after 5 cycles and examination of the testes, epididymides, accessory sex glands, and plasma hormone levels after 6 cycles of the seminiferous epithelium.

If an agent is shown to alter male reproduction in a test extending over 6 cycles of chronic exposure (Test 1 or Test 2 as described under protocols for testing), it may be desirable to determine if the effect is reversible (Test 3). A test of reversibility should extend over 18 cycles of the seminiferous epithelium. Chronic exposure to the agent should extend over 6 cycles, and 12 cycles should elapse after the termination of exposure to allow for restoration of normal reproductive function.

Although the recovery period in man is usually longer, these animal data should provide a clear indication if complete recovery will occur in man (compare radiation data of Meistrich et al. [13] in the mouse and Rowley et al. [14] in man).

Evaluation of Reproductive Damage in Exposed or Potentially Exposed Men

General

Two types of studies in humans seem particularly relevant to the objectives of a male reproduction risk assessment. The first involves surveillance studies, in which periodic checking is done on men in a setting (e.g., industrial or agricultural) that might, in the future, involve the risk of a reproductive defect. An example of such a setting would be a chemical company in which substances are prepared that are known from animal studies to cause reproductive toxicity when administered in high dosage but not at a dosage up to 10 times that expected for human exposure. The safety factor may be variable, however, and depends on the quality of the animal study from which it was derived. This type of surveillance is important for at least two reasons: (a) the sensitivity of men may be greater than allowed for by the tenfold safety factor and (b) the exposure of the workers may be greater than originally estimated. The methods for surveillance of this type could be quite innocuous and could be incorporated into an annual medical checkup if this were already a practice.

The second type of study would be of men who have been or are being exposed to a known reproductive toxin in dosages likely to be toxic in man as based on animal studies. This type of study could be used in men exposed to high dosages of one or more general toxins for which the effect on testicular function had not been studied carefully in animals.

Surveillance studies

Men could be asked yearly whether they have been attempting to cause a pregnancy and have been unable to do so. The prevalence of infertility in couples within the reproductive age group is approximately 15% (74). If more than 20% of men between 19 and 35 have been unable to produce a pregnancy in over one year of *unprotected* intercourse, a possible toxic effect should be looked for in a rigorous manner as outlined in the following section on known toxic exposure.

Testicular length could be measured on annual physical examination. If the distribution of testicular size for men falls significantly below the lower norm (3.5 cm for Caucasian and Black) for that age group and ethnic background (76), a toxic effect should be suspected.

Blood levels of follicle-stimulating hormone could be measured yearly. If mean levels significantly vary from those of age-matched controls, a toxic effect should be suspected.

If any of these three variables suggest testicular toxicity, a more detailed study of the population should be undertaken, as outlined below.

Study of men with known toxic exposure

Where a human population is suspected of being at reproductive risk because of environmental hazards, a number of potentially toxic agents may be involved, and the duration and level of exposure may vary within the population. Although each potential toxicant should be carefully tested by the laboratory screening methods outlined in this document, it would be useful to make a more immediate and direct assessment of fertility potential in the exposed population. The requirements for this include capacity for rapid response to the subjects, feasibility, sensitivity, and data that can be analyzed statistically. The data obtained in such studies should provide an initial indication of the degree of testicular damage, and where an environmental reproductive hazard has been identified, more detailed studies may be undertaken to characterize objectively male reproductive dysfunction.

To carry out these studies, a specialized team and a modest amount of equipment would be needed. The latter could be installed at locally available facilities, or a mobile laboratory could be equipped. Detailed medical, reproductive, and occupational histories should be taken from each exposed subject and a physical examination given. At least five semen samples should be evaluated per individual at two-day intervals. Objective data on testicular size and consistency could be obtained by sonography and tonometry. Blood and urine could be obtained at this time for endocrine studies and/or toxicant levels. Controls to be studied must be carefully chosen and matched. Before a national data base is established, individuals should be selected according to epidemiological advice. For the details of these analyses, see "Study of men with known toxic exposure" in the Appendix to this chapter.

Statistically significant differences between the exposed and the control groups (matched for age, occupation, geographical location) in seminal fluid and blood hormone measurements would be evidence for an effect of the exposure on male reproductive function. An adverse effect would be expected to decrease sperm counts, motilities, and numbers of sperm with normal morphology; if the effect were sufficiently severe, blood testosterone levels would decrease. If the toxic effects were directly on the testis (as is the case with the great majority of known toxins), follicle-stimulating hormone (FSH) levels would increase. With a mild toxic effect on the testis, blood FSH levels after administration of gonadotropin-releasing hormone (GnRH) might exceed normal responses, even when basal FSH levels are normal. If the toxic effect were primarily on the pituitary gland or central nervous system, luteinizing hormone (LH) and FSH levels would tend to decrease.

If not established initially (Surveillance studies, v. sup.), other comparisons between the exposed and control groups should include (a) rate of infertility as indicated by the number of men who have not been able to induce a pregnancy in over one year of intercourse without using contraceptives, and (b) testicular size, with particular attention to the number of men with testicular length less than 3.5 cm.

Differences between the exposed and control groups in these last two assessments, suggested also for the initial screen, will be found when reproductive toxicity is sufficiently severe. However, measurements of fertility and testicular size would be expected to be less sensitive in revealing mild defects in gonadal function than the seminal fluid and blood hormone measurements described above.

Additional comment on human testing procedures

Blood samples for hormone measurement and noninvasive procedures such as testicular length may be the more feasible parameters to evaluate because of the added difficulty in obtaining semen samples, in some human populations at least. However, where these give equivocal results, it is likely that semen analyses will help to resolve the fundamental dilemma.

An elevated FSH level is a sensitive indicator of decreased function of the germinal epithelium in man and experimental animals. However, while there is no doubt that increased FSH levels usually imply decreased sperm production (9, 14, 21, 77, 78), measuring FSH levels is probably a less dependable test than direct sperm counts, for it is a consistent marker only of severe oligozoospermia or azoospermia (53, 79, 80). Measurements of FSH seem useful adjuncts to sperm counts, therefore, and indicators of the direct action of toxic agents on pituitary function. Despite their wide variability in man, total sperm per ejaculate are usually a *more sensitive* measure of testicular damage than elevated FSH levels.

Comprehensive semen analysis requires an assessment of sperm morphology as well as total sperm per ejaculate. This aspect of the human ejaculate has received considerable general comment as a parameter that also often falls below the standards that might be expected for animals living in the same area. Since about 30% of the spermatozoa are abnormal in semen from a presumed fertile group of men, only by using large groups of 100 or so persons would it be possible to detect increases in abnormal spermatozoa of the order of 10% in cross-sectional studies in which only one to four samples are collected for each man in exposed and control groups. Despite the relatively variable morphology of a significant proportion of spermatozoa in the human ejaculate, sperm morphology tends to be fairly constant for one individual (81). This justifies the use of fewer men in longitudinal studies where such studies can be undertaken (as compared to postexposure analyses), since the men can then act as their own controls (81).

Human sperm morphology classification is currently subjective, personality oriented, and nonstandard (82). However, detailed "type classification" (i.e., oval versus tapering versus amorphous) may not be required to identify groups of individuals at reproductive risk. In normal fertile human semen, sperm morphology is relatively uniform, more than 50% of the sperm having the typical "oval" shape. In contrast, infertile human semen is characterized by a diversity of abnormal sperm sizes and shapes. If objective, morphometric data describing sperm size and shape (e.g., head length, width, area, and circumference; tail midpiece width) were obtained from individuals at potential risk, these could be compared statistically with data from the matched control group. Significantly greater dispersion in the morphometric parameters of the exposed group might indicate increased reproductive dysfunction in the population. The magnitude of differences between the exposed group and the control group might also provide an indication of the severity of testicular damage. As noted earlier, the methods for automatic evaluation of sperm morphology are not well established and need considerable refinement and validation (6).

Assessment of risk to men

Assessment of risk to reproductive performance and fertility in men is inadequately tested at present. The quantitative assessment of risk to general human health from exposure to environmental toxicants has been approached by relating the probable or estimated dose of a suspect toxic agent to the occurrence of deleterious effects on the basis of either epidemiologic data on human populations or of experimental data from animal studies. It seems likely that threshold effects will appear for most agents. Ideally, assessment of the effects of these agents upon male reproductive function should be based upon human epidemiologic data. However, there are few epidemiologic risk assessment data regarding the effect of environmental agents on the fertility of men. Thus, at present a quantitative risk assessment must depend on extrapolation to man of measurements of the reproductive end points in experimental animal systems discussed here. One approach to risk assessment estimates the acceptable daily intake (ADI) of a chemical, defined as the exposure level that is anticipated to be without risk to the species. It should be cautioned that the ADI represents only a judgment, is not an estimate of risk nor a guarantee of absolute safety, and is subject to modification as additional relevant information becomes available.

To account for the uncertainties involved in extrapolating from animals to man, the ADI includes an uncertainty or safety factor to the highest no-adverse-effect level measured in an animal study. A no-adverse-effect level is defined here as a dose for which no significant difference is found between control and treated animals for any of the end points measured adequately. It is important that a statistically significant effect also be biologically significant. This uncertainty factor will depend on (a) the animal species/strain; (b) the quality of the experimental data; (c) the availability of comparative pharmacokinetic information on the animal species' and man's absorption, distribution, metabolism, binding, and elimination of the chemical; and (d) any other relevant comparative information on structurally similar chemicals. In the absence of these comparative data, we should follow the guidelines of the Safe Drinking Water Committee, National Research Council of the National Academy of Sciences (83), and recommend an arbitrary uncertainty factor of 100 for adequate animal studies. In the case of human male reproduction, the size of this factor seems more than justified by increasing evidence that the human testis functions less efficiently and possibly closer to a point of pathology than that of the animal models recommended (2, 7, 8). Thus, for an agent causing a reversible action in a model animal, the ADI would be 0.01 times the no-adverse-effect level for the most sensitive criterion and the most sensitive species evaluated, whether rat or rabbit. A daily exposure or intake above this level represents a risk of reproductive damage to human males. For irreversible effects on male reproductive function, we feel we can make no recommendation for a quantitative risk assessment.

Protocols for Testing Compounds with Animal Models

The actual criteria to be evaluated in each test are shown in Table 8. The time schedules for conducting Tests 1, 2, and 3 are shown in Table 11. If pharmacological studies show that the test compound may bioaccumulate so that the body burden increases beyond an interval equal to one cycle of the seminiferous epithelium, the treatment interval of both Test 1 and Test 2 must be increased appropriately. At least 5 cycles should elapse after reaching maximum body load.

Test 1 — initial screen

As an initial screening procedure, animal exposure will be greater than or equal to half of a maximum tolerated dose ($\geqslant$0.5 MTD) of the test agent for an interval equal to 6 cycles of the germinal epithelium. An initial screen using an acute exposure is considered to be unnecessary, because the subchronic test is more sensitive.

To initially assess risk to male reproduction, a compound should be subjected to *in vivo* tests utilizing both rats and rabbits. A compound producing no statistically significant alteration in any criterion for either species when given at $\geqslant$0.5 MTD would be considered to be safe for humans (see safety factor in risk assessment). A statistically significant alteration in any criterion would necessitate conduct of a Test-2 evaluation to establish a dose-response curve, unless manufacture or use of the agent were to cease, or if a larger safety factor were used. Test 1 (Tables 8 and 11) uses both rats and rabbits and is detailed in the Appendix to this chapter. The fixed time schedule is designed to maximize the probability of detecting any decrease in reproductive function.

Test 2 — dose response curve

1. The general approach used in the initial screen (Test 1) will be used except that additional criteria of reproductive damage are included (Table 7). The dose-response curve will include at least three points, usually the dose used in Test 1, and −1 and −2 log doses and must extend down to the human exposure level (if known) or until no statistically significant response is obtained in any test. Both 0-dose and untreated controls could be included to detect effects of handling that might be associated with agent administration. If necessary, additional tests will be run to attain these end points. Both rats and rabbits must be used. The fixed time schedule (Table 11) is essential to measure accurately the extent of damage to

TABLE 11 Chronology of Conduct for Test with Animal Models
(Expressed as Day of Study)

Test	Rat	Rabbit
Test 1 or 2[a]		
Condition males	$-21 \to 0$	$-28 \to 0$
Obtain preexperimental body weight	$-14 + 0$	$-14 + 0$
Evaluate preexperimental semen	NA[b]	$-14 \to 0$
Initiate compound administration	day 0	day 0
Continue compound administration	$0 \to 77$	$0 \to 64$
Weigh weekly	$0 \to 78$	$0 \to 65$
Collect experimental semen (each 3–4 days)	NA	$3–4 \to 53–54$
Measure testis size weekly	NA	$0 \to 65$
Expose to females or artifically inseminate females	$65 \to 71$	$54 \to 57$
Sexually rest males	$71 \to 78$	$58 \to 65$
Kill males	78	65
Kill females	$83 \to 89^c$	NA
Allow females to kindle	NA	$85 \to 90$
Test 3[a]		
Condition males	$-21 \to 0$	$-28 \to 0$
Obtain preexperimental body weight	$-7 + 0$	$-7 + 0$
Evaluate preexperimental semen	NA	$-14 \to 0$
Initiate compound administration	0	0
Continue compound administration	$0 \to 77$	$0 \to 64$
Collect experimental semen	NA	$35 \to 64$
	NA	$118 \to 140$
	NA	$158 \to 194$
Expose to females or artifically inseminate females	$215 \to 221$	$184 \to 187$
Kill 1/3 of males	78	64
1/3 of males	155	128
1/3 of males	232	193
Kill females 18–24 hours past mating	$216 \to 222$	NA
12–18 days past mating	233	NA
Allow females to kindle	NA	$215 \to 218$

[a]Rats will be weighed weekly. Rabbits will be weighed weekly, testis size measured weekly, and semen will be collected twice weekly (every 3 to 4 days). Schedule is for a compound that does not accumulate for a long time; steady state level in body tissues reached in $<10–12$ days.

[b]NA = not applicable.

[c]Kill females 18 days after mating, as determined by a vaginal smear.

the different aspects of male reproductive function and to enable a prediction of human risk.

2. In evaluating testicular histology, sections representing at least two loci will be used. The diameter of 50 tubules will be measured; the percentage of seminiferous tubule cross-sections ($N = 250$) having mature spermatids lining the tubule lumen and the percentage of

tubules (N = 250) devoid of germ cells other than spermatogonia will be determined. Evaluations of the morphology of sperm in the cauda epididymidis and ejaculated semen will be more comprehensive than in Test 1. The serum concentrations of luteinizing hormone (LH), FSH, and testosterone also will be determined.

Test 3 — recovery study

1. Test 3 is a long-term study designed to test the reversibility of damage to male reproduction and also to evaluate sperm transport, penetration of sperm into ova, and early embryonic death. Many agents that cause degeneration of the germinal epithelium and azoospermia will not damage the stem spermatogonia. If the latter remain, eventual recovery of the germinal epithelium is likely. This test measures recovery of the germinal epithelium and fertility, at 6 cycles and 12 cycles (155 days for rats and 128 days for rabbits) after ending a 6-cycle exposure to the test compound. Although recovery of the germinal epithelium might not be complete by 12 cycles after exposure, some onset of recovery probably should be detectable by then if it will occur eventually. If the test compound is one known to bioaccumulate, longer treatment periods (as used in Test 2) and recovery periods (at least twice the duration of the treatment period) are essential.

2. The criteria evaluated (Tables 8 and 11) are the same as those in Test 2, except that data on fertilized rat eggs are necessary. Consequently, each male will be exposed to four female rats. Two females will be killed 18 to 24 hours after mating (as determined by the presence of vaginal plugs) and ova recovered by flushing. The two other female rats will be killed 12 to 18 days after mating. Measurement of concentrations of the compound in blood and seminal plasma at steady state are desirable, since these data may be useful in predicting potential damage in humans and the prognosis for recovery from such damage.

3. The time schedule (Table 11) for conduct of the study could be modified by extending the treatment beyond 6 cycles, but the timing of evaluations between days 215 and 233 for rats and days 184 and 218 for rabbits may not need to be altered.

4. Complete reversibility is considered to be restoration, to at least 90% of control levels at 12 cycles after cessation of exposure, of *all* criteria adversely altered in males after 6 cycles of exposure (in Test 2 or Test 3) at a given dose.

Research Needed

Until about 15 years ago only outline information about the male tract was available (84–86). Although much precise data has appeared since then for the animal models suggested and even some for man (65, 87, 88), it is difficult to compare the two. Research into this and related aspects as suggested below is a critical element for establishment of a reliable assay and evaluation of risk in males.

1. Variance components for characteristics of semen (total volume, total sperm per ejaculate, percentage of motile sperm, and incidence of sperm abnormalities) are available for rabbits (see Table 10) but have not been reported for man. This information should be obtained for men of different age groups (<20, 21–30, 31–40, >40) with different life styles or occupations, so that efficient and meaningful evaluations can be made.

2. The influence of an abstinence interval on characteristics of human semen should be evaluated critically for men of 20 to 30, 30 to 40, and >40 years of age. Procedures for reducing the influence of an abstinence interval on estimates of sperm production (e.g., normalization of data for each ejaculate by dividing by the number of days of abstinence) should be evaluated. It is also unclear what effect repeated ejaculation has on the absolute concentrations of many seminal compounds that might be measured as indicators of the activity of accessory glands in man or the amount of the test agent in seminal plasma.

3. For the human, the relationship should be determined among testicular size, tonometric measurements or testicular consistency, and sperm output as well as other ejaculate characteristics.

4. Relationships need to be established among testicular histology, ejaculate characteristics, sperm morphology, and fertility of humans, rabbits, and rats. Indices of fertility should be calculated.

5. Automatic or semiautomatic morphometric procedures should be further developed for analysis of the morphology of human spermatozoa and spermatozoa from test animals. First-generation systems for automated evaluations are available (e.g., at Lawrence Livermore Laboratory), but the instrumentation and software need additional refinement and validation before these techniques can be applied routinely in analyses of human sperm morphology (89, 90).

Sperm morphometry can be obtained for living sperm cells or from stained seminal smears, by methods becoming increasingly automated, either using flow cytometry (89) or tracing sperm shape from the screen of a video monitor using an electronic planimeter-digitizer integrated into a minicomputer (49). The use of sperm morphology for diagnosis or prognostication of specific reproductive disorders will require a "type classification" of individual sperm abnormalities. The determination of such a classification can be made by computer on the basis of the morphometric data obtained. Research should be encouraged to develop such computer software. A classification system based on morphometric standards should be developed.

6. A data bank should be established for (a) the control data from screening tests with animals to build a large base for computation of variations associated with each characteristic among trials, locations, season, year, etc.; (b) the chemical nature of compounds tested and found in an initial screen to damage some aspect of male reproduction or to have no effect; and (c) the chemical nature of all compounds found to have a deleterious effect on male reproduction, the nature, extent, and incidence of damage in each exposure dose, and interval to recovery.

7. Available data on effects of agents known to alter human male reproduction should be correlated with data on their action in test animals in a battery of tests. The repeatability and relative sensitivity of the tests within and between species should be determined. Recommendations for specific studies are as follows:

(a) Obtain more extensive and accurate analytical data on semen from men exposed to chemotherapy and the effects of parallel levels of chemotherapy in animals.

(b) Bring together existing radiation studies in human and experimental animals for development of models in which to base chemical risk assessment data.

(c) Obtain better data in experimental animals on effects of dibromochloropropane or other agents known to be harmful to man.

8. The relative usefulness of basal FSH concentration in blood or of FSH response to GnRH as indicators of testicular damage should be compared with seminal analyses to determine their sensitivity (see Table 10 and Appendix to this chapter). For screening of large numbers of human males, it would be useful to know the single most sensitive index of testicular toxicity. In man, a test based on a blood sample is more practical than one requiring submission of a seminal fluid sample.

9. The responsiveness of Leydig cells should be evaluated. Well-characterized *in vitro* bioassays for LH have been developed. Rat or mouse Leydig cells are incubated over several hours with various concentrations of LH. The amount of testosterone produced by the Leydig cells is measured. A potential testicular toxin could be studied by exposing it, in various concentrations, with LH to the

Leydig cell preparations and comparing the amount of testosterone produced to that produced by cells exposed to LH alone.

10. The responsiveness of Sertoli cells should be evaluated. Sertoli cell cultures, preferably from postpubertal males, can be used. The production of known secretory products, such as transferrin or androgen-binding protein, following stimulation by FSH, can be measured as an index of their activity. An effect of a toxin would be reflected in that index. A major question is the relationship of *in vitro* toxicity to *in vivo* toxicity, particularly considering the short-term nature of the tests and the long-term nature of *in vivo* exposure. However, some of the *in vitro* tests provide limited opportunity to evaluate human tissue directly with animal models.

11. Competitive mating (heterospermic insemination) should be evaluated as a screening assay. The use of a mixed-insemination assay (91–93) for screening toxicants offers a means of increasing the sensitivity of fertilization assays and should be explored. Rabbits and possibly rats could be used. Semen from exposed and control males would be mixed and inseminated into the same female and the paternity of the offspring established by genetic markers (i.e., eye or coat color). This has good potential for use as a screening assay of superior sensitivity which could simultaneously assess disturbances of sexual behavior, sperm quality, sperm transport in the female, fertilization, and embryonic and fetal development. A limited number of trials with the system should be adequate to determine its utility.

12. The direct assessment of damage to the sperm genome would permit routine screening and monitoring of males for exposure in the workplace to chemicals that may be hazards to their reproductive capacity. Further studies might attempt the following:

(a) Establish the degree of correlation between abnormal sperm head morphology and an aberrant chromosome complement.

(b) Develop sensitive methods for the identification and measurement of alkylated or modified DNA bases.

(c) Improve the methodology to quantitate alkylated amino acids, since there is evidence that alkylation of sperm chromatin proteins also contributes to reproduction failure.

(d) Develop methods to detect damage to sperm chromatin (e.g., enzymatic detection of strand breaks in sperm DNA).

Additional studies could be designed and sponsored to evaluate the suitability of the four techniques discussed above as routine procedures for detection of genetic abnormalities by direct observation of spermatozoa and of the male pronucleus.

REFERENCES

1. Smith, K. D., Rodriguez-Rigau, L. J. and Steinberger, E.: Relation between indices of semen analysis and pregnancy rate in infertile couples. Fertil. Steril. 28: 1314–1319, 1977.

2. Amann, R. P.: A critical review of methods for evaluation of spermatogenesis from seminal characteristics. J. Androl. 2: 39–60, 1981.

3. Barfield, A., Melo, J., Coutinho, E., Alvarezs, F., Faundes, A., Brache, V., Leon, P., Frick, J., Bartsch, G. and Weiske, W. H.: Pregnancies associated with sperm concentrations below 10 million-ml in clinical studies of a potential male contraceptive method, monthly depot medroxyprogesterone acetate and testosterone esters. Contraception 20(2): 121–127, 1979.

4. David, G., Jouannet, P., Martin-Boyee, A., Spira, A. and Schwartz, D.: Sperm counts in fertile and infertile men. Fertil. Steril. 31(4): 453–455, 1979.

5. Zuckerman, Z., Rodriguez-Rigau, L. J., Weiss, D. B., Chowdhury, A. K., Smith, K. D. and Steinberger, E.: Quantitative analysis of the seminiferous epithelium in human testicular biopsies and the relation of spermatogenesis to sperm density. Fertil. Steril. 30: 448–455, 1978.

6. Freund, M.: Standards for the rating of human sperm morphology. Int. J. Fertil. 11: 97–180, 1966.

7. Johnson, L., Petty, C. S. and Neaves, W. B.: A comparative study of daily sperm production and testicular composition in humans and rats. Biol. Reprod. 22: 1233–1243, 1980.

8. Amann, R. P. and Howards, S. S.: Daily spermatozoal production and epididymal spermatozoal reserves of the human male. J. Urol. 124: 211–215, 1980.

9. Smith, K. D. and Steinberger, E.: What is oligospermia? In: The Testis in Normal and Infertile Men, D. Troen and H. Nankin, Eds., Raven Press: New York; pp. 489–503, 1977.

10. Salisbury, G. W., Van Demark, N. L. and Lodge, L. R.: Physiology of reproduction and artificial insemination of cattle, W. H. Freeman and Co.: San Francisco; 788 pp., 1978.

11. MacLeod, J., Hotchkiss, R. S. and Sitterson, B. W.: Recovery of male fertility after sterilization by nuclear radiation. J. Am. Med. Assoc. 187: 637–641, 1964.

12. Amelar, R. D., Dubin, L. and Hotchkiss, R. S.: Restoration of fertility following unilateral orchiectomy and radiation therapy for testicular tumors. J. Urol. 106: 714–718, 1971.

13. Meistrich, M. L., Hunter, N., Suzuki, N., Trostle, P. K. and Withers, H. R.: Gradual regeneration of mouse testicular stem cells after ionizing radiation. Radiat. Res. 74: 349–362, 1978.

14. Rowley, M. J., Leach, D. R., Warner, G. A. and Heller, C. G.: Effect of graded doses of ionizing radiation on human testes. Radiat. Res. 59: 665–678, 1974.

15. Cheviakoff, S., Calamera, J. C., Morgenfield, M. and Mancini, R. E.: Spermatogenesis in patients with lymphoma after treatment with chlorambucil. J. Reprod. Fertil. 33: 155–157, 1973.

16. Sherins, R. J. and DeVita, V. T., Jr.: Effect of drug treatment for lymphoma on male reproductive capacity—studies of men in remission after therapy. Ann. Intern. Med. 79: 216–220, 1973.

17. Sieber, S. M. and Adamson, R. H.: Toxicity of antineoplastic agents in man: chromosomal aberrations, antifertility effects, congenital malformations, and carcinogenic potential. Adv. Cancer Res. 22: 57–155, 1975.

18. Lu, C. C. and Meistrich, M. L.: Cytotoxic effects of chemotherapeutic drugs on mouse testis cells. Cancer Res. 39: 3575–3582, 1979.

19. Torkelson, T. R., Sadele, S. E., Rowe, V. K., Kodama, J. K., Anderson, H. H., Loquvam, G. S. and Hine, C. H.: Toxicologic investigations of 1,2-dibromo-3-chloropropane. Toxicol. Appl. Pharmacol. 3: 545–559, 1961.

20. Whorton, M. D., Krauss, R. M., Marshall, S. and Milby, T. H.: Infertility in male pesticide workers. Lancet 2(8051): 1259–1261, 1977.

21. Glass, R. I., Lyness, R. N., Mengle, D. C., Powell, K. E. and Kahn, E.: Sperm count depression in pesticide applicators exposed to dibromochloropropane. Am. J. Epidemiol. 109(3): 346–351, 1979.

22. Lantz, G. D., Cunningham, G. R., Huckins, C. and Lipshultz, L. I.: Recovery from severe oligospermia after exposure to dibromochloropropane. Fertil. Steril. 35: 46–53, 1981.

23. Amann, R. P.: Use of animal models for detecting specific alterations in reproduction. Appl. Fund. Toxicol.; in press, 1982.

24. Amann, R. P.: Sperm production rates. In: The Testis, Vol. 1, A. Johnson, W. Gomes, and N. Van Demark, Eds., Academic Press, Inc.: New York; pp. 433–482, 1970.

25. Carson, W. S. and Amann, R. P.: The male rabbit. VI. Effects of ejaculation and season on testicular size and function. J. Anim. Sci. 32: 302–309, 1972.

26. Foote, R. H.: Research techniques to study reproductive physiology in the male. In: Techniques and Procedures in Animal Science Research. American Society of Animal Producers: Albany, New York; pp. 81–100, 1969.

27. Robb, G. W., Amann, R. P. and Killian, G. J.: Daily sperm production and epididymal sperm reserves of pubertal and adult rats. J. Reprod. Fertil. 54: 103–107, 1978.

28. Amann, R. P. and Lambiase, J. T.: The male rabbit. III. Determination of daily sperm production by means of testicular homogenates. J. Anim. Sci. 28: 369–374, 1969.

29. Amann, R. P., Kavanaugh, J. F., Griel, L. C., Jr. and Voglmayr, J. K.: Sperm production of Holstein bulls determined from testicular spermatid reserves, after cannulation of rete testis or vas deferens, and by daily ejaculation. J. Dairy Sci. 57: 93–99, 1974.

30. Johnson, L., Petty, C. S. and Neaves, W. B.: A new approach to quantification of spermatogenesis and its application to germinal cell attrition during human spermiogenesis. Biol. Reprod. 25: 217–226, 1981.
31. Clermont, Y.: Kinetics of spermatogenesis in mammals: seminiferous epithelial cycles and spermatogonial renewal. Physiol. Rev. 52: 198–236, 1972.
32. Swierstra, E. E. and Foote, R. H.: Cytology and kinetics of spermatogenesis in the rabbit. J. Reprod. Fertil. 5: 309–322, 1963.
33. Swierstra, E. E., Whitefield, J. W. and Foote, R. H.: Action of amphotericin B (fungizone) on spermatogenesis in the rabbit. J. Reprod. Fertil. 7: 13–19, 1964.
34. Berndtson, W. E.: Methods for quantifying mammalian spermatogenesis: a review. J. Anim. Sci. 44: 819–833, 1977.
35. Lu, C. C., Meistrich, M. L. and Thames, H. D.: Survival of mouse testicular stem cells after gamma or neutron irradiation. Radiat. Res. 81: 402–415, 1980.
36. Amann, R. P.: The male rabbit. IV. Quantitative testicular histology and comparisons between daily sperm production as determined histologically and daily sperm output. Fertil. Steril. 21: 662–672, 1970.
37. Lambiase, J. T., Jr. and Amann, R. P.: The male rabbit. V. Changes in sperm reserves and resorption rate induced by ejaculation and sexual rest. J. Anim. Sci. 28: 542–549, 1969.
38. Fray, C. S., Hoffes, A. P. and Fawcett, D. W.: Reexamination of motility patterns of rat epididymal spermatozoa. Anat. Rec. 173: 301–308, 1972.
39. Gaddum, P.: Sperm maturation in male reproductive tract—development of motility. Anat. Rec. 161: 471–482, 1968.
40. Blandau, R. J. and Rumery, R. E.: Relationship of swimming movements of epididymal spermatozoa to their fertilizing capacity. Fertil. Steril. 15: 571–579, 1964.
41. Lock, L. F. and Soares, E. R.: Increases in morphologically abnormal sperm in rats exposed to ^{60}Co irradiation. Environ. Mutagen. 2: 125–131, 1980.
42. Harasymowyez, J., Ball, L. and Seidel, G. E., Jr.: Evaluation of bovine spermatozoal morphologic features after staining or fixation. Am. J. Vet. Res. 37: 1053–1057, 1976.
43. Holtz, W. and Foote, R. H.: Anatomy of reproductive system in male Dutch rabbits *(Oryctolagus cuniculum)* with special emphasis on the accessory sex glands. J. Morph. 158: 1–20, 1978.
44. Amann, R. P.: Effect of ejaculation frequency and breed on semen characteristics and sperm output of rabbits. J. Reprod. Fertil. 11: 291–293, 1966.
45. Holtz, W. and Foote, R. H.: Sperm production, output, and urinary loss in the rabbit. Proc. Soc. Exp. Biol. Med. 141: 958–962, 1972.
46. Kirton, K. E., Desjardins, C. and Hafs, H. D.: Levels of some normal constituents of rabbit semen during repetitive ejaculation. Fertil. Steril. 17: 204–211, 1966.

47. Paufler, S. K. and Foote, R. H.: Effect of triethylenemelamine (TEM) and cadmium chloride on spermatogenesis in rabbits. J. Reprod. Fertil. 19: 309–319, 1969.
48. Schwartz, D., Laplanche, A., Jouannet, P. and David, G.: Within-subject variability of human semen in regard to sperm count, volume, total number of spermatozoa, and length of abstinence. J. Reprod. Fertil. 57: 391–395, 1979.
49. Katz, D. F. and Overstreet, J. W.: Sperm motility assessment by videomicrography. Fertil. Steril. 35(2): 188–193, 1981.
50. Eliasson, R.: Analyses of semen. In: Progress in Infertility, S. J. Behram and R. W. Kistnes, Eds., Little Brown and Co.: Boston; pp. 691–713, 1975.
51. Holtz, W. and Foote, R. H.: Composition of rabbit semen and the origin of several constituents. Biol. Reprod. 18: 286–292, 1978.
52. Baker, M. W. G., Bremner, W. J., Burger, H. G., de Kretser, D. M., Dulmanis, A., Eddie, L., Hudson, B., Keogh, E. J., Lee, V. W. K. and Rennie, G.: Testicular control of FSH secretion. Rec. Prog. Horm. Res. 32: 429, 1976.
53. de Kretser, D. M., Kerr, J. B., Rick, K. A., Risbridger, G. and Dobas, M.: Hormonal factor involved in normal spermatogenesis. In: Testicular Development, Structure, and Function, A. Steinberger and E. Steinberger, Eds., Raven Press: New York; pp. 109–115, 1980.
54. Psychoyos, A.: Hormonal control of ovoimplantation. Vitam. Horm. 31: 201–256, 1973.
55. Bedford, J. M.: Techniques and criteria used in the study of mammalian fertilization. In: Methods in Mammalian Embryology, J. C. David, Ed., W. H. Freeman and Co.: San Francisco; pp. 37–63, 1971.
56. Yanagimachi, R., Yanagimachi, H. and Rogers, B. J.: Use of zona-free animal ova as a test system for assessment of fertilizing capacity of human spermatozoa. Biol. Reprod. 15(4): 471–476, 1976.
57. Hahn, J., Foote, R. H. and Cranch, E. T.: Tonometer for measuring testicular consistency of bulls to predict semen quality. J. Anim. Sci. 29: 483–489, 1969.
58. Oakberg, E. F.: Degeneration of spermatogonia of the mouse following exposure to X-rays, and stages in the mitotic cycle at which death occurs. J. Morph. 97: 39–54, 1955.
59. Nicander, L.: Studies on the regional histology and cytochemistry of the ductus epididymis in rabbits. Acta Morphol. Neerl. Scand. 1: 99–118, 1957.
60. Reid, B. L. and Cleland, K. W.: The structure and function of the epididymis. I. The histology of the rat epididymis. Aust. J. Zool. 5: 223–246, 1957.
61. Brooks, D. E.: Biochemical environment of sperm maturation. In: The Spermatozoon: Maturation, Motility, Surface Properties and Comparative Aspects, D. W. Fawcett and J. M. Bedford, Eds., Urban and Schwarzenberg: Baltimore; pp. 23–34, 1979.
62. Brandes, D., Ed.: Male Accessory Sex Organs. Academic Press: New York; 527 pp., 1974.

63. Hammerstedt, R. H.: Characterization of sperm surfaces using physical techniques. In: Spermatozoon: Maturation, Motility, and Surface Properties and Comparative Aspects, D. W. Fawcett and J. M. Bedford, Eds., Urban and Schwarzenberg: Baltimore; pp. 205–216, 1979.

64. Bedford, J. M. and Cooper, G. W.: Membrane fusion events in the fertilization of vertebrate egg. In: Cell Surface Reviews, Vol. 5, Membrane Fusion, Elsevier North Holland: Amsterdam; pp. 66–111, 1978.

65. Mann, T. and Lutwak-Mann, C.: Male Reproductive Function and Semen, Springer-Verlag: New York; 495 pp., 1981.

66. Hammerstedt, R. H.: Monitoring the metabolic rate of germ cells and sperm. In: Reproductive Processes and Contraception, K. W. McKerns, Ed., Plenum Publishing: New York; pp. 353–391, 1981.

67. Hegde, U. C., Shastry, P. R. and Rao, S. S.: Use of dithiothreitol for improved visibility of F-body in human Y-bearing spermatozoa. J. Reprod. Fertil. 53: 403–405, 1978.

68. Evenson, D. P., Darzynkiewicz, Z. and Melamed, M. R.: Relation of mammalian sperm chromation heterogeneity to fertility. Science 210: 1131–1133, 1980.

69. Gledhill, B. L., Lake, S. and Dean, P. N.: Flow cytometry and sorting of sperm and other male germ cells. In: Flow Cytometry and Sorting, M. Melamed, P. Mullaney, and M. Mendelsohn, Eds., J. Wiley and Sons: New York; pp. 471–484, 1979.

70. Rudak, E., Jacobs, P. A. and Yanagimachi, R.: Direct analysis of chromosome constitution of human spermatozoa. Nature 274: 911–913, 1978.

71. Aafjes, J. H., Vels, J. M. and Schenck, E.: Fertility of rats with artificial oligozoospermia. J. Reprod. Fertil. 58(2): 345–352, 1980.

72. Desjardins, C., Kirton, K. T. and Hafs, H. D.: Sperm output of rabbits at various ejaculation frequencies and their use in the design of experiments. J. Reprod. Fertil. 15: 27–32, 1968.

73. Seidel, G. E., Jr. and Foote, R. H.: Variance components of semen criteria from bulls ejaculated frequently and their use in experimental design. J. Dairy Sci. 56: 399–405, 1973.

74. MacLeod, J.: Human male infertility. Obstet. Gynecol. Surv. 26: 335–351, 1971.

75. Janick, J. and MacLeod, J.: Measurement of human spermatozoan mobility. Fertil. Steril. 21: 140–146, 1970.

76. Lubs, H. A.: Testicular size in Kleinfelter's Syndrome in men over fifty. Report of a case with XXY/XY mosaicism. New Engl. J. Med. 267: 326–331, 1962.

77. Asbjornsen, G., Molne, K., Klepp, O. and Aakvaag, A.: Testicular function after combination chemotherapy for Hodgkin's disease. Scand. J. Haematol. 16(1): 66–69, 1976.

78. Van Thiel, D. H., Sherins, R. J., Meyers, G. H. and Devita, V. T., Jr.: Evidence for a specific seminiferous tubular factor affecting follicle-stimulating hormone secretion in man. J. Clin. Invest. 51: 1009–1019, 1972.

79. Cunningham, G. R. and Huckins, C.: Serum FSH, LH, and testosterone in ^{60}Co γ-irradiated male rats. Radiat. Res. 76: 331–338, 1978.

80. Verjans, H. L. and Eik-Nes, K. B.: Hypothalamic-pituitary-testicular system following testicular X-irradiation. Acta Endorcinol. 83(1): 190–200, 1976.

81. MacLeod, J.: Human seminal cytology following the administration of certain antispermatogenic compounds. In: Agents Affecting Fertility, C. R. Austin and J. S. Perry, Eds., Little Brown and Co.: Boston; pp. 93–123, 1965.

82. Belsey, M. A., Eliasson, R., Gallegos, A. J., Maghissi, K. S., Paulsen, C. A. and Prasad, M. R. N.: Laboratory Manual for the Examination of Human Semen and Semen-Cervical Mucus Interaction, Press Concern: Singapore; 43 pp., 1980.

83. National Academy of Sciences: Drinking Water and Health, Vol. 3, National Academy Press: Washington, D.C.; pp. 25–265, 1980.

84. Young, W. C., Ed.: Sex and Internal Secretions, Vol. 1, 3rd Edition, Williams and Wilkins: Baltimore; pp. 161–448, 1961.

85. Young, W. C., Ed.: Sex and Internal Secretions, Vol. 2, 3rd Edition, Williams and Wilkins: Baltimore; pp. 707–796, 1173–1239, 1961.

86. Mann, T.: The Biochemistry of Semen and of the Male Reproductive Tract, Methuen: London; 240 pp., 1964.

87. Hamilton, D. W. and Greep, R. O., Eds.: Handbook of Physiology, Section 7, Vol. 5: Male Reproductive System, American Physiological Society: Washington, D.C.; 519 pp., 1975.

88. Greep, R. O., Koblinsky, M. A. and Jaffee, F. S., Eds.: Reproduction and Human Welfare: A Challenge to Research, MIT Press: Cambridge, Mass.; 622 pp., 1976.

89. Wyrobek, A. J. and Gledhill, B. L.: Human semen assays for workplace monitoring. In: Proceedings of Workshop on Methodology for Assessing Reproductive Hazards in the Workplace. Center for Disease Control, National Institute for Occupational Health and Safety; pp. 327–355, 1980.

90. Gledhill, B. L. Personal communication, Lawrence Livermore Laboratory: California; 1981.

91. Beatty, R. A., Bennett, G. H., Hall, J. G., Hancock, J. L. and Stewart, D. L.: An experiment with heterospermic insemination in cattle. J. Reprod. Fertil. 19: 491–502, 1969.

92. Overstreet, J. W. and Adams, C. E.: Mechanisms of selective fertilization in the rabbit: sperm transport and viability. J. Reprod. Fertil. 26: 219–231, 1971.

93. O'Connor, M. T., Amann, R. P. and Saacke, R. G.: Comparisons of computer evaluations of spermatozoal motility with standard laboratory tests and their use for predicting fertility. J. Animal Sci.; in press, 1981.

APPENDIX

DETAILS OF TEST PROTOCOLS AND GLOSSARY OF TERMS FOR MALE RISK ASSESSMENT

I. DESCRIPTION AND DISCUSSION OF TESTS USEFUL IN ANIMAL MODELS OR MAN

Body Weight

Measure body weight of all test animals weekly starting two weeks before administration of the compound and continuing until termination of the study.

Testicular Characteristics

Testis size in situ

The number of spermatozoa, and to a lesser extent the quantity of testosterone, produced by the testes of normal individuals is a function of testis size and, to a lesser extent, of variation in the proportion of the testis composed of germinal elements and interstitial tissue (1). Therefore, assessment of testicular size is very important from a functional standpoint. In scrotal animals, testicular size can be measured easily, accurately, repeatedly and without damage to the individual (2–5). In many species of laboratory and domestic animals, testis size is correlated (correlation coefficient r = 0.8–0.9) with sperm output in ejaculated semen when males are ejaculated frequently (e.g., four ejaculates per week) (1, 2). Changes in testis size should be correlated with results of other tests to increase the accuracy of the analysis.

Measurements of testis size should be made biweekly or weekly with animal models and could be made part of an annual physical examination given to men working in a hazardous environment.

Scrotal circumference. This measurement can be taken easily in animals with pendulous scrotum (4). To reduce variation, the measurements should be made with a standard procedure.

Linear measurements. Length and width can be measured in species such as dogs, rabbits, bulls, and horses (1, 2–5). Length and width measurements are correlated with testis weight ($\geq$0.90). If these data are correlated with seminal characteristics, adjustment for time lag in spermatogenesis and sperm transport through the excurrent ducts is necessary.

Testis weight

Each testis must be dissected free from the epididymis and pampiniform plexus, and weighed when model animals are killed or castrated. Testis weight, relative to norms for that breed or strain, can reveal gross differences resulting from a treatment.

Spermatid reserves

Counting of homogenization-resistant spermatid nuclei in testicular homogenates is a simple, accurate, and sensitive method for measuring sperm production. This method can be accomplished with simple equipment and does not require extensive training. The nuclei of elongated spermatids are resistant to mechanical and chemical disruption and are easily identified after physical disruption of testicular tissue (1, 6, 7). With human testes, small biopsies can be used (8), and the tissue should be fixed in glutaraldehyde before homogenization, because some spermatid nuclei may not be fully condensed (9). The interval from when spermatids acquire the resistance to homogenization until spermiation is a constant for a species or strain (1). Thus, the number of resistant spermatids is a direct measure of the production of spermatozoa by the testis and the survival of the precursor spermatogenic cells (1).

Either biopsy material (20 mg or more), a representative sample taken at necropsy, or the entire testes (for rats and rabbits) can be homogenized or disrupted ultrasonically (6, 10). Resistant spermatid nuclei are counted in a cytometer (at least 6 chambers per sample). Counts should be expressed on both a per-testis basis and a per-mg-of-parenchyma basis (11). Counts from treated animals should be compared to those for concurrent control males.

The time of this analysis relative to an acute treatment or the onset of chronic treatment can be varied so as to reveal possible damage to cells in specific stages of spermatogenesis. The interval between onset of treatment and evaluation should be expressed in terms of the duration of one "cycle of the seminiferous epithelium" for that species. Preferred times for evaluating agents should be chosen according to the kinetics of spermatogenesis (7, 12–17).

Histopathological analysis of testes

Histologic analyses of testicular biopsies or whole testes must be performed on animal models and, in special cases, could be performed on man. Qualitative and quantitative analyses of increasing complexity yield general or precise information. It is axiomatic that serious disturbance will be evident to the observer using direct simple evaluations of germinal epithelium in histological preparations of whole testes. Threshold effects require a detailed evaluation such as that recommended below. Electron microscopy is not considered to be useful for screening of damaging agents. Testicular tissue must be fixed immediately in Bouin's or Zenker's fluid (10% formalin is *not* satisfactory). Slides should be stained with hematoxylin and eosin for simple analyses and with periodic-acid-Schiff-hematoxylin if a more precise determination of the stages of spermatids is required (17).

Gross morphology. Appearance of Leydig interstitial cells (18); occurrence of lymphoid cell or macrophage infiltration (19); presence of germ cells of each stage (spermatogonia, spermatocytes, spermatids, sperm) in seminiferous tubules (20); presence of large numbers of degenerating (21), multinucleate (22), or abnormal germ cells (23) should be noted.

Nonfunctional tubules. The percentage of tubular cross-sections with *no evidence of spermatogenesis* (i.e., <4 germ cells) should be scored during brief examination at 100X or 400X magnification of 250 cross-sections per testis (24, 25). Such examination could be performed 2 to 7 days after acute treatment or 6 cycles after onset of chronic treatment. The integrity of the layer of Sertoli cells in these sterile tubules should also be noted.

Tubules with spermatids lining the lumen. The end product of spermatogenesis is reflected in the "mature" spermatids about to be released from the Sertoli cells. Tubules with spermatids aligned at the lumen can be easily recognized (16). The incidence of such tubules is a characteristic of the species. Deviations between control and treated males reflect testicular dysfunction.

Seminiferous tubule diameter. Diameters can change with interference of tubular function (26). Measurements of minor diameter should be taken on essentially round tubule cross-sections (cut at right angles to their long axis) taken from several different locations in sections used for scanning other aspects of gross histology. Only tubules in which the minor diameter is within 10% of the major diameter (i.e., the sections are essentially transverse) should be measured.

Counts of preleptotene or leptotene spermatocytes

The number of leptotene spermatocytes per Sertoli cell with a visible nucleolus can be quantitated because of a characteristic nuclear morphology of leptotene spermatocytes (27, 28). The number of leptotene spermatocytes and the number of Sertoli cells with a visible nucleolus should be determined in the same set of tubules. The ratio of spermatocytes per Sertoli cell is a sensitive measure of testicular damage; effects of as little as 5 rad of radiation can be detected (20).

Epididymal Characteristics

Weight of distal half of epididymis

The distal portion of the epididymis can be isolated by severing the corpus epididymidis midway between the caput and cauda and at the junction of the distal cauda with the ductus deferens. The distal epididymis and the contralateral epididymis should be weighed promptly.

Number of sperm in the distal half of epididymis

One epididymis, weighed as above, is homogenized to liberate the spermatozoa contained therein (6, 7); simple mincing of the tissue is inadequate. Sperm cells are counted using a cytometer (at least 6 chambers counted per sample). The results should be expressed as total counts. The epididymis evaluated could be alternated within each control or treated group to ensure representative sampling if there is any systematic difference between sides.

Motility of sperm from the distal end

Sperm from the distal end of the remaining cauda epididymidis will be expressed into a phosphate-buffered saline solution containing 5 mM of glucose or pyruvate plus 0.1% bovine serum albumin, polyvinyl alcohol, or similar macromolecules. Sperm concentration should be standardized to 10×10^6 to 40×10^6 per ml, and the percentage of motile sperm determined at 37°C under conditions similar to those described for estimating percentage of motile spermatozoa in ejaculated semen.

Gross morphology of spermatozoa from the distal end

The same semen preparation used for estimating the percentage of motile spermatozoa will be viewed by phase-contrast microscopy at 400X for evaluation of gross morphology. The proportion of the spermatozoa from treated animals, in comparison with controls, with misshapen heads, acrosomal defects or distorted swimming patterns, will be estimated.

Detailed morphology of spermatozoa from the distal end

For detailed evaluation of sperm morphology, smears will be prepared by a procedure minimizing artifacts (29), then stained with eosin-nigrosin (or other differential stain). A total of 200 to 400 spermatozoa should be classified per sample. Smears can be preserved as a permanent record, or videotapes can be prepared. Detailed morphological or morphometric examination is possible with either.

Accessory Sex Gland Characteristics

1. The accessory sex glands are biomonitors of androgen production by the testes. Thus, accessory sex gland weight will be recorded when each male animal is killed.

2. For rats, the vesicular glands are discrete organs and very easily distinguishable. After removal and expression of the viscid fluid, the glands should be blotted and weighed.

3. The individual accessory sex glands are not discrete in the rabbit (30). Thus, the total set of accessory glands will be excised as a single unit, blotted, and weighed. The organs will be reweighed after removal of any secretion present in the vesicular glands.

Seminal Analysis

General aspects of seminal analysis

(a) Analysis of semen offers a convenient approach for monitoring function of the germinal epithelium and, with less specificity, the functions of the epididymides, prostate, vesicular glands, and bulbourethral glands (11). An abnormality in epididymal function may be detected in semen ejaculated 3 to 15 days after epididymal dysfunction. An abnormality in spermatogenesis typically cannot be detected in semen until after at least 1 to 4 cycles of the seminiferous epithelium (16—64 days in man or 11—43 days in rabbit) have passed (1, 11, 14, 31), plus time for epididymal transport. This long interval is required because an agent must accumulate to a toxic concentration and produce a lesion in germ cells at a specific point in their development (often >2 cycles of the seminiferous epithelium before the end of spermatogenesis) before production of more mature germ cells is affected. After passage of a given interval, evidence of the lesion can be seen within the testis, but the lesion will not be evident in semen until the affected germ cells have completed spermatogenesis (2—3 cycles), passed through the epididymis (4—16 days), and appeared as spermatozoa in ejaculated semen.

(b) Multiple samples can and should be obtained from each individual male. Both quantitative and qualitative characteristics of more than one ejaculate must be evaluated to gain a reasonable understanding of testicular function (1, 11, 32). Data for samples collected before experimental exposure can be used as one basis for assigning males to control or treatment groups or as a covariant in the statistical analysis.

(c) The species, strain, and age of males; testicular size; season; method of semen collection; and interval since the previous ejaculation(s) all influence quantitative characteristics of semen and must be carefully controlled (11, 33).

(d) If seminal analyses are planned, use of a species from which semen can be collected by artificial vagina or digital manipulation (masturbation) is essential. Suitable species include man, rabbit, dog, bull, and minipig (1, 2, 11, 32—34). The rabbit is the species of choice for screening potentially toxic agents because of size, availability, cost, and ease of use. Small rabbits (e.g., Dutch Belted) are as good as larger breeds (e.g., New Zealand White) and are cheaper to house. Rams, goats, and stallions are less ideal because seasonal changes are more profound. Subhuman primates probably will not be used frequently because of their limited numbers and cost. Although useful in many other aspects, rats have limited use (as do mice) because of their small seminal volume, difficulty in quantifying seminal characteristics, and the necessity to use electro-stimulation for semen collection. Improved procedures for quantitative collection of semen from rats or mice are unlikely to overcome their limitations. However, as outlined above, cauda epididymal sperm can be obtained (on a one-time basis) from a mouse or rat and evaluation of the motility and morphology of epididymal sperm is desirable.

(e) For most studies, sexually mature males (body weight $\leqslant 90\%$ of maximum value for that strain) should be used. If consequences of exposure before puberty are to be evaluated, the age or body weight when a given number of sperm are first ejaculated may be a useful criterion (requires at least weekly testing) and the postpubertal changes in semen quality could be monitored (33).

By monitoring seminal characteristics longitudinally from exposure, through a reasonable interval when an effect might be expressed (6 X the duration of the cycle of the seminiferous epithelium for the species studied) and during a recovery phase (if appropriate) of twice this duration, information can be obtained on the point when damage is expressed and when recovery occurs (1, 2, 14).

Volume

(a) Volume of the ejaculate should be measured with an accuracy of greater than 90 to 95%. To measure accurately ejaculates with a small volume, it is recommended that collection tubes be preweighed and ejaculate volume be calculated from the weight, assuming a specific gravity of 1.0.

(b) Systematic errors associated with seminal loss during collection or transfer to a measuring device should be minimized. Measurement of ejaculate volume within the collection vessel, after addition of a known volume of buffer if essential, is desirable. Systematic errors in measurement often can be corrected for (1, 2, 11).

(c) If a uniform collection interval and standardized collection procedure are used (1, 11), differences of $>25\%$ in ejaculate volume probably could be detected in a longitudinal study utilizing ten rabbits per treatment group (35). A difference of this magnitude probably would reflect abnormal function of the accessory sex glands if unaccompanied by a change in sperm output.

(d) The coefficient of variation for volume of a human ejaculate is unknown but could be calculated from available data. It is likely that a sizable number of ejaculates must be evaluated for each individual in a group to detect a 25% change in seminal volume.

Seminal plasma constituents

(a) The biochemical components of seminal plasma may reflect the functionality of the epididymides and accessory sex glands (11), but the concentration of a compound in a seminal plasma has limited diagnostic value (11).

(b) If collection procedures are rigidly standardized for a species, a marked change ($>25\%$) in the total mass of a constituent ejaculated, could reflect the function of the excurrent duct system or one or more accessory sex glands. It is not clear at present, however, whether any constituents change their concentration markedly in the course of repeated ejaculations with humans (see Research Needed).

Spermatozoal concentration

(a) The term spermatozoal *concentration* is preferred to those of sperm count or sperm density.

(b) Sperm concentration, by itself, provides little information (11), but sperm concentration must be determined accurately so that the total number of sperm per ejaculate can be calculated (see below).

(c) Sperm concentration should be determined using a calibrated spectrophotometer or electronic cell counter, if contaminating cells or debris are not a problem, because of their accuracy and precision (2, 11). If extraneous material is present in the semen, visual counts using a cytometer are essential. Use of a cytometer (with a phase-contrast microscope) is time consuming, and $\geqslant 6$ replicate counts are necessary to achieve $\geqslant 90\%$ accuracy for a single sample.

Total sperm per ejaculate

(a) The term total number of sperm per ejaculate (volume X sperm concentration) is preferable to that of total sperm count.

(b) Total sperm per ejaculate represents the number of sperm coming from the excurrent duct system and is independent of the degree of dilution by accessory sex gland fluid (11).

(c) When semen is collected by a uniform procedure and total sperm per ejaculate is averaged over time, daily sperm output (number of sperm in a series of ejaculates divided by the time span) can be calculated. Daily sperm output, in rabbits and bulls, is highly correlated ($\cong 0.9$) with daily sperm production (1, 11, 36).

(d) To measure daily sperm output accurately (1, 11), a uniform interval of one, two, or three days between semen collections is essential, and the series of ejaculates should extend over 14 (preferably 20) days (data for the first 3–6 ejaculates should be excluded a priori and data for the remaining >6 samples averaged).

(e) If semen is collected infrequently (one ejaculate weekly), a 50% reduction in sperm production probably would be undetectable (11). To have a 75% chance of detecting a difference of 50% daily sperm output would require about 20 rabbits per treatment and ejaculation for >5 weeks (35).

(f) A formula relating the coefficient of variation (CV) between counts; the significance level at which the statistical test is to be performed, α (e.g., $\alpha = 0.05$, $\alpha = 0.01$); the desired power or sensitivity of the statistical test, 1-β (e.g., 1-β = 0.50, 1-β = 0.90); and the sample size of the study, N (i.e., N treated and N control animals), to the required change (in terms of percent of 'normal' or control values) in the test criteria is given by

$$\frac{(Z_\alpha + Z_{1-\beta})(CV)}{\sqrt{N/2}} = \% \text{ change}$$

where Z_α = 1.645 for α = 0.05 and Z_α = 2.326 for α = 0.01, and $Z_{1-\beta}$ = 0, 0.253, 0.524, 0.842, and 1.281 for 1-β = 0.5, 0.6, 0.7, 0.8, and 0.9, respectively. It should be noted that this formula assumes a one-sided statistical test, that is, looking for changes between treated and control animals in only one direction (e.g., decrease in sperm concentration). Along with the coefficients of variation given in Table 10, it can be used to determine the adequacy of different experimental designs. For example, the largest coefficient of variation, other than for accessory sex gland weight, is for the test criterion total sperm/ejaculate in Dutch Belted rabbits, CV = 0.75. Assuming that any statistical comparison between 12 treated and 12 control rabbits is conducted at the α = 0.05 level (i.e., 5% test level), to have at least a 50% chance of detecting a statistically significant difference (i.e., power = 0.50), then the treatment must produce at least a 50% change in the test criterion, that is, (1.654 + 0)(0.75)/$\sqrt{12/2}$ = 0.5. Because each of the other criteria, except for accessory sex glands, have coefficients of variation of less than 0.75, they would have the same power, 50%, of detecting a smaller effect; for example, for testis weight, CV = 0.2 giving a percent change of 13%, (1.645 + 0) (0.20)/$\sqrt{12/2}$ = 0.13.

Sperm motility

(a) Rigid control of temperature at 37°C and other conditions of evaluation are essential (2, 11).

(b) Visual evaluation of sperm motility using diluted semen and a phase-contrast microscope is informative and rapid, although subjective. Visual estimations are adequate for an initial screen, provided that control and treatment samples are presented randomly in a blind manner to the observer. For second- or third-level analysis, more objective procedures, such as videotape and analyses or track motility (37–39) should be considered.

(c) The percentage of progressively motile sperm, the translatory velocity, and the presence of sperm moving in a circular pattern or backward should be recorded.

(d) A reduced percentage of motile sperm might reflect abnormal spermatogenesis, abnormal functions of the epididymis or entrance of an antimotility factor into the semen (via the excurrent ducts, prostate, bulbourethral glands, or vesicular glands) where it could exert a direct effect on the sperm.

(e) The percentage of motile sperm probably reflects both normality of spermatogenesis and sperm metabolism.

(f) Variation within males in the percentage of motile spermatozoa (and probably velocity) is less than for ejaculate volume or total sperm per ejaculate (35, 40).

(g) A significant decrease in the percentage of motile sperm would be a strong indicator for a potential decline in fertility and especially so if sperm numbers are limited.

Spermatozoal morphology

(a) Abnormalities of sperm morphology reflect dysfunction of the germinal epithelium (primary abnormality) or of the excurrent duct system (secondary abnormality). Certain abnormalities cannot be clearly attributed to a specific site of action.

(b) An increase in the percentage of abnormal sperm may precede a decline in the total number of sperm per ejaculate (if any) and can serve as a sensitive indicator of epididymal or testicular function.

(c) Within a male, sperm morphology is quite consistent over time (41). This consistency makes sperm morphology a sensitive probe while requiring fewer samples per male for an experiment of a given precision.

(d) Evaluation of sperm morphology is subjective (42) and must be carefully standardized among laboratories (11, 42, 43). A detailed classification probably is unnecessary in an initial screening process. Classification of spermatozoa, based on light microscopy, as normal or abnormal head, normal or abnormal tail is adequate for a screen. For second- or third-level screening, a more complex classification might be used (42–44).

(e) Evaluation of sperm morphology using wet preparations and phase-contrast microscopy is recommended for simplicity and freedom from artifacts (11, 29), although preparation and retention of stained smears (a simple stain like eosion-nigrosin or eosin-analine blue) is desirable for archival purposes.

Ejaculated sperm as an *in vitro* test system

(a) Substances can pass from blood into semen via the fluid from the excurrent ducts and accessory sex glands and could be spermicidal or alter sperm function.

(b) Agents can be screened economically by incubating sperm *in vitro* under standard conditions in a protein-containing buffer at 37°C for 4 to 8 hours. Sperm could be exposed to the agent briefly (10–30 minutes) or throughout the incubation period. A dose-response curve should be established using objective methods of evaluation and sperm from humans or other species (rats, rabbits, dogs, or bulls).

(c) The decline in percentage of motile sperm over time is an excellent criterion, but other criteria (e.g., integrity of the acrosome and plasma membrane, oxygen consumption, adenosine 5'-triphosphate content, or degree of agglutination [45]) could be used.

(d) Compounds that are spermicidal *in vitro* at concentrations that could be anticipated or shown to be present in blood or seminal plasma should be carefully screened *in vivo*. Failure to demonstrate a spermicidal action *in vitro* is *not* evidence that an agent would be free of effects on male reproduction, nor is spermicidal action *in vitro* evidence of *in vivo* activity.

Assessment of Male Reproductive Toxicity
Using Endocrinological Methods

General

(a) This section describes general aspects of applying endocrinological methods to the study of male reproduction. Specific applications of these techniques to studies in animals and men are described elsewhere in this account.

Normal male reproductive function requires hormonal stimulation of the testes and production by the testes of adequate numbers of sperm and the hormone testosterone. Luteinizing hormone (LH) and follicle-stimulating hormone (FSH) are the two hormones necessary to maintain normal testicular function. These hormones originate in the pituitary gland and travel through the blood to affect the testis. The production of LH and FSH and their release from the pituitary are stimulated by gonadotropin-releasing hormone (GnRH), which is produced in the hypothalamus at the base of the brain. Testosterone and other hormones produced by the testis are carried by the blood throughout the body. At the pituitary, these hormones tend to decrease the production of LH and FSH, that is, they exert a "negative feedback" effect on LH and FSH secretion.

(b) If a defect occurs in hypothalamic or pituitary function, blood levels of FSH and LH will tend to decrease.

(c) If a defect occurs in the testis (either in sperm or testosterone production), FSH and LH levels will tend to *increase* because of lack of the "negative feedback" effect of testicular hormones.

(d) In addition to its effects on the pituitary, testosterone exerts many effects throughout the body. It is necessary for expression of male sexual behavior and the ability to perform intercourse, stimulates muscle and bone development and red blood cell production, and is essential for many other aspects of normal body function. A decrease in blood levels of testosterone can be expected to affect all these functions adversely.

(e) It is clearly established in all mammalian species investigated that an endocrine defect in the brain, pituitary, or testis may inhibit spermatogenesis and normal sexual behavior and cause sterility. Less severe defects in these tissues (not so severe as to lead to infertility) might be detected by measurements of hormone concentration in the blood. In certain situations, including studies of human beings, hormone measurements are very practical, because they can be performed on ordinary samples of blood serum, whereas seminal fluid or testicular tissue may be difficult or impossible to obtain.

(f) Hormonal measurements are important and sensitive tools in the assessment of toxicity to the male reproductive system. They can be compared directly among a variety of species and between control and treated groups of any species including man. Hormonal data may give a clue as to the tissue in which a toxic effect is occurring.

Hormone assay and application

(a) Hormones commonly are measured by radioimmunoassay. This is an extremely sensitive technique and, when done in a competent laboratory, is quite reliable for measuring testosterone, FSH, and LH. Many commercial laboratories perform radio-immunoassays for LH, FSH, and testosterone in human blood samples.

Developing these assays requires familiarity with the technique, access to counters for radioactivity and availability of specialized assay reagents such as purified preparations of the hormones and antibodies to these hormones.

(b) Testosterone is an identical molecule in all species, so it can be measured from any species in a single assay. Nevertheless, appropriate species controls are essential to preclude the possibility that a cross-reacting molecule is altering test results. Both LH and FSH are protein hormones that differ slightly in molecular structure among species. Assays for LH and for FSH tend to be species-specific, so that assay reagents appropriate for the species in question generally are required for measuring LH or FSH. For rats and man these reagents are widely available, and such reagents have recently been introduced for rabbits. For normal adult male rats, however, the concentration of LH in peripheral blood is usually below the sensitivity level of available radioimmunoassays.

Measurement of blood levels of hormones yields a direct assessment of the level of exposure necessary to produce a toxic effect. The methodology is sufficiently accurate to detect changes of 20% in mean hormone levels using generally available numbers of animals (e.g., 20 per group). Statistical adequacy for these assays when performed competently is very good; in general, within-assay coefficients of variations are below 10%, and between-assay coefficients of variations are less than 15% (46). These assays are specific measures of reproductive toxicity; disease of other organ systems will not affect these measurements unless the disease concomitantly affects the reproductive system.

Any statistically significant difference between hormone levels in a comparison of control and exposed animals or men can be accepted as strong evidence for a toxic effect of the exposure on reproduction. If such an effect were established by animal studies, this could be used as strong evidence that a similar effect would occur in human beings. In essentially every instance studied in detail, agents found to be testicular toxins in one species have a similar effect in other species (47).

(c) Hormone levels may be measured in single blood samples, although evaluation of several samples taken at two-hour intervals is better. The time of day should be standardized because of diurnal rhythms. Ordinarily, no special preparation is necessary concerning diet or physical activity.

(d) For all known reproductive toxins, the damage to reproduction is reversible if the exposure level is so low as to produce only a minimally detectable effect. With a more severe insult or a prolonged toxin exposure, the damage may be irreversible.

Examination of Known Toxic Exposures

Humans

Seminal fluid analyses. At least one and preferably five seminal fluids obtained by masturbation at two-day intervals should be submitted by each man. Precautions must be taken to ensure an accurate measurement of seminal volume (11). The age of the individuals and the abstinence interval between samples should also be considered in the evaluation (48–50). Variability among ejaculates from the same individual is influenced by the length of abstinence (50). The semen should be analyzed for volume, sperm concentration, and total sperm per ejaculate. Total sperm per ejaculate must be calculated and compared with norms. Sperm motility (at 37°C) should be objectively assessed using phase-contrast microscopy; motility should be characterized in terms of percentage of motility and velocity. If feasible, videotapes should be made of the living sperm cells, with the tapes being subsequently analyzed in a laboratory familiar with this technique. Seminal smears should be fixed (29) for subsequent analysis. Tests of sperm function such as penetration of zona-free hamster eggs may not be feasible for field work. However, if persistent infertility remains undiagnosed after completion of the other studies proposed, the hamster egg *in vitro* penetration test (51) should be considered.

Blood hormone levels. Peripheral venous blood samples should be obtained at a standardized time of day (preferably 0700–0900 hours) for measurement of serum luteinizing hormone (LH), follicle-stimulating hormone (FSH), and testosterone by radioimmunoassay. Hormone measurements on both the exposed and control groups should be performed in the same laboratory. This laboratory must be one that is recognized for reliability and that maintains careful quality control records.

Gonadotropin-releasing hormone (GnRH) test. This test has been demonstrated to be capable of detecting mild degrees of primary testicular dysfunction insufficient to elevate basal hormone levels out of the normal range (52). It is not necessary if the basal, unstimulated-hormone levels are abnormal. Blood samples for measurement of LH and FSH are obtained before and at 30, 60, and 90 minutes after administration of GnRH (100 μg i.v.). Synthetic GnRH is now available for use as an investigational new drug through several pharmaceutical companies and will probably be approved by the Food and Drug Administration for general use.

Animal models

Rats. Twenty mature male rats of a highly fertile strain (body weight must be >90% of adult normal for that strain) will be given ⩾0.5 of the maximum tolerated dose (MTD) by inhalation, intraperitoneal (i.p.) injection, drinking water, or gavage for a period of exactly 6 cycles of seminiferous epithelium (12.9 days per cycle X 6 = 77 days). An appropriate control group (or groups) will be evaluated concurrently. If the agent is given by injection or gavage, both nonhandled and vehicle-injected control groups are necessary. Each rat will be weighed weekly starting 14 days prior to initial dosing (day −14) and continuing to day 78. Each male will be caged with two sexually mature, virgin female rats between days 65 and 71 (for a total of 6 nights) to evaluate fertility. On day 78, blood will be taken by cardiac puncture immediately (<1 minute) after removing a male rat from his cage in the animal room and the male rat killed. Serum will be frozen.

Both testes will be weighed. One will be fixed in Bouin's fluid for histologic examination and determination of the number of leptotene spermatocytes per Sertoli cell nucleolus. The second testis will be homogenized and the number of resistant spermatid nuclei determined. The vesicular glands will be weighed as an indirect measure of circulating testosterone concentration. The distal half of one epididymis (half corpus plus cauda) will be weighed. Spermatozoa will be expressed from the severed end of the distal cauda epididymidis into phosphate-buffered saline containing 0.1% bovine serum albumin. The percentage of progressively motile spermatozoa will be determined under phase-contrast microscopy and the incidence of abnormal spermatozoa recorded. A stained slide of the spermatozoa will be made for documentation. The distal half of the contralateral epididymis will be isolated, homogenized, and the total number of sperm heads determined. Concentration of testosterone, LH, and FSH in serum will be determined.

The females will be killed on day 83 to 89 (18 days after mating), and the numbers of corpora lutea and implantation sites, as well as embryo viability, will be determined.

Rabbits. Twelve mature male rabbits (body weight must be ⩾90% of adult normal for that strain) will be given the ⩾0.5 MTD by inhalation, i.p. injection, or in drinking water (the same route of administration should be used for both rats and rabbits when possible) for a period of 6 cycles of seminiferous epithelium (10.7 days per cycle X 6 = 64 days). An appropriate control group (or groups) will be established concurrently. Testis size and body weight will be measured weekly starting on day −14 and continuing through day 65. Two ejaculates will be collected every 3 to 4 days (e.g., Monday and Thursday) using an artificial vagina. The volume, with and without gel, concentration, and total sperm per ejaculate will be measured. Sperm motility and gross sperm morphology will be determined using phase-contrast microscopy. Libido will be subjectively assessed weekly. Each male will be mated with two virgins, sexually mature females over a 4-day period (between days 54 and 57) and the females allowed to kindle. On day 65, blood will be taken by cardiac puncture and the male rabbits killed. Evaluation will be similar to that for rats. Testis size and weight, number of homogenization resistant spermatids, weight and sperm content of the distal epididymis, and motility and morphology of sperm from the distal epididymis will be evaluated. Gross histologic evaluation and enumeration of the number of leptotene spermatocytes per Sertoli cell nucleolus will be made on one testis fixed in Bouin's fluid. Weight of the accessory sex glands will be recorded as an indirect measure of circulating-testosterone level. Blood will be saved for possible assay for FSH, LH, and testosterone.

Pregnancy rate and litter size will be determined for females bred to each male.

Fertility Testing

Tests available

Humans. *In vitro* oocyte penetration tests are the only means available for assessing the fertilizing capacity of human sperm. Since human *in vitro* fertilization cannot itself be used as a test, substitutes must be used for the human ovum. These include the zona pellucida of stored human follicular oocytes (53) and the zona-free hamster vitellus (54). Regrettably, these tests have not been carefully validated to establish variation among independent analyses of the same ejaculate or of different ejaculates from one male. In situations where *in vitro* testing of human sperm fertility is indicated, the use of a double-fluorescent-label competitive sperm penetration assay with the zona-free hamster egg will increase the sensitivity of the test (55). The sensitivity of the hamster egg penetration assay is also increased by attempting to count the total number of sperm per penetrated hamster vitellus as well as the percentage of penetrated eggs.

Animals. *In vivo* mating tests should be carried out with laboratory rats and rabbits. A visible reduction of quality of the ejaculate may not be reflected in the fertility level because of a superfluidity of spermatozoa in the ejaculate. The sensitivity of the test can be increased greatly by insemination with critical numbers of sperm (ca. 1×10^6 to 2×10^6 in the case of the rabbit). *In vitro* tests are unnecessary for use with animals.

Usefulness

The animal tests are useful since they measure the ability of sperm to reach and fertilize an ovum. The *in vivo* tests are well established and reliable if critical sperm numbers are used. Tests of the fertilizing capacity of human sperm allow assessment of semen from a human population at reproductive risk when the hazard being studied has produced fertilization dysfunction in the animal tests. If fully validated, the *in vitro* human fertilization system also could be used to determine the dose-response relationship of a compound to the fertility of human sperm.

Sensitivity

Although simple mating trials with evaluation of offspring provide some useful information on fertilization, this is an all-or-none measurement. Since sperm production is greatly in excess of that required for fertility, significant reductions in sperm output by the testes may not be detectable by this method (2). The test can be improved as an assay of fertilization ability by using artificial insemination with sperm in limited numbers. Another potentially useful approach involves competition between two populations of spermatozoa from males whose status in relation to each other is known, with expectation of change in the competitive relations following exposure of the male to an agent of interest (39). This latter approach requires further validation (see Research Needed).

In fertility tests embryos should be recovered as early as the 2–8 cell stage. Evaluation of a second group of pregnant rats between days 15 and 19 enables comparison of the numbers of viable and dead embryos with the number of corpora lutea and is more efficient than allowing parturition. If rabbit eggs of 2–8 cells are recovered, the number of sperm associated with fertilized and unfertilized eggs can be counted. This should bring to light abnormalities in sperm transport or abnormalities of cleavage that may result from defects in the sperm genome (see Sperm Nucleus Integrity).

Specificity

The fertilization tests are specific indicators of reproductive toxicity, although they have limited value in the broader context of toxicological testings. The toxicological end points in the *in vivo* animal fertilization system include failures of (a) sperm-egg association, (b) sperm penetration of the zona pellucida, and (c) normal cleavage of the early embryo. All of these events are directly analogous to those occurring in humans. A consistent failure of human spermatozoa to penetrate >10% of zona-free hamster eggs probably reflects an abnormality of the physiological events associated with fertilization (i.e., sperm capacitation and/or the acrosome reaction). These events are presumed to be the same as those required for human fertilization *in vivo*.

Sperm Nucleus Integrity

A toxic chemical may cause infertility of exposed males through action on the sperm genome rather than by alteration of the normal course of spermatogenesis. Thus, the usual parameters used to assess semen quality will not detect this cause of infertility. Genetic damage to the spermatozoa is best assessed by mating the exposed male to untreated females and observing the progeny for sterility, heritable translocations, sex-chromosome loss, specific locus mutations, mutations affecting the skeleton and eye, and dominant lethality. These procedures are covered in the U.S. Environmental Protection Agency's proposed Guidelines for Mutagenicity Risk Assessment (56). Of these tests, only dominant lethality has a bearing on the fertility of an exposed male. This effect can be detected by evaluation of fertilized eggs and embryos as outlined in the section titled Fertility Testing.

Since the animal tests referred to above are not applicable to the human male, it would be desirable to be able to assess the genetic integrity of human spermatozoa directly. Four methods for the detection of chromosomal abnormalities in spermatozoa are as follows:

Quinacrine staining for Y-chromosome aneuploidy

This technique, used also by inference for possible somatic chromosome aneuploidy (57), is easy and economical, does not require sophisticated equipment, and should be suitable for the study of population groups. However, the method is subject to many errors, and its accuracy has been questioned (58, 59). The reliability of the procedure can be improved by using more rigid criteria for scoring fluorescent Y bodies (60). Nevertheless, the technique's reliability has not been sufficiently established to warrant its use as a routine screening procedure.

Spermatozoal morphology

Chemicals, radiation, heat, and a variety of insults increase the proportion of morphologically abnormal sperm in the ejaculate, and an increase in the number of abnormal sperm usually results in impaired fertility. This aspect has been considered in the section on evaluation of semen quality. That these abnormalities are associated with chromosomal damage, however, has not been demonstrated.

Karyotyping of human spermatozoa by the denuded-hamster-egg technique

This procedure is technically difficult, requires highly trained personnel, and at present should be reserved for evaluation of those cases where additional evidence that chromosome abnormalities are a factor in reduced fertility is desired.

Genetic damage with consequences for male fertility also can arise from strand breaks, base alterations, and base substitution in the sperm DNA. Except for strand breaks, methods are currently unavailable for the detection of these lesions. Future work to develop qualitative and quantitative procedures for the detection of such lesions in sperm DNA would be desirable, since sperm with an apparently normal chromosome complement may be responsible for male fertility problems.

Dose Response

1. The criteria for evaluating male reproductive processes, discussed above, can be quantified. In most cases, the procedures are objective, accurate, precise, and sensitive. Data for each criterion have a considerable response span, although values for normal individuals may not have a normal distribution.

2. A number of agents acting on the reproductive system are known to induce a partial suppression in one or more of the criteria listed when given in low dosages and a more severe effect as the dose is increased.

3. It is likely that separate dose-response curves can be established for several criteria with each agent tested. The sensitivity of a particular test would depend upon the nature of the agent.

4. It is likely that agents affecting reproduction have a threshold dose below which damage does not occur.

5. It is unlikely, however, that chronic administration of an agent at $\geqslant 0.5$ MTD would not induce a detectable alteration in one or more of the criteria listed, in at least one of two species, if the agent in fact has a deleterious effect on reproductive function in the human male.

6. Reversibility of damage to the male reproductive system often occurs after exposure to the causative agent is terminated. Complete regeneration repair usually will require an interval equivalent to at least three to four and often more than six to twelve cycles of the seminiferous epithelium.

REFERENCES

1. Amann, R. P.: Sperm production rates. In: The Testis, Vol. 1, A. Johnson, W. Gomes, and N. Van Demark, Eds., Academic Press, Inc.: New York; pp. 433–482, 1970.
2. Foote, R. H.: Research techniques to study reproductive physiology in the male. In: Techniques and Procedures in Animal Science Research, American Society of Animal Producers: Albany, New York; pp. 81–100, 1969.
3. Carson, W. S. and Amann, R. P.: The male rabbit. VI. Effects of ejaculation and season on testicular size and function. J. Anim. Sci. 34:302–309, 1973.
4. Coulter, G. H. and Foote, R. H.: Bovine testicular measurements as indicators of reproductive performance and their relationship to productive traits in cattle: a review. Theriogenol. 11:297–311, 1979.
5. Paufler, S. K., Van Vleck, L. D. and Foote, R. H.: Estimation of testicular size in live rabbits. Int. J. Fertil. 14:188–191, 1969.
6. Amann, R. P. and Lambiase, J. T.: The male rabbit. III. Determination of daily sperm production by means of testicular homogenates. J. Anim. Sci. 28:369–374, 1969.
7. Robb, G. W., Amann, R. P. and Killian, G. J.: Daily sperm production and epididymal sperm reserves of pubertal and adult rats. J. Reprod. Fertil. 54: 103–107, 1978.
8. Johnson, L., Petty, C. S. and Neaves, W. B.: The relationship of biopsy evaluations and testicular measurements to overall daily sperm production in human testes. Fertil. Steril. 34: 36–40, 1980.
9. Johnson, L., Petty, C. S. and Neaves, W. B.: A new approach to quantification of spermatogenesis and its application to germinal cell attrition during human spermiogenesis. Biol. Reprod. 25: 217–226, 1981.

10. Mian, T. A., Suzuki, N., Glenn, H. J., Haynie, T. P. and Meistrich, M. L.: Radiation damage to mouse testis cells from ^{99}M technetium pertechnetate. J. Nucl. Med. 18: 1116–1122, 1977.

11. Amann, R. P.: A critical review of methods for evaluation of spermatogenesis from seminal characteristics. J. Androl.; in press, 1981.

12. Lu, C. C., Meistrich, M. L. and Thames, H. O., Jr.: Survival of mouse testicular stem cells after gamma or neutron irradiation. Radiat. Res. 81: 402–415, 1980.

13. Meistrich, M. L., Hunter, N., Suzuki, N., Trostle, P. K. and Withers, H. R.: Gradual regeneration of mouse testicular stem cells after ionizing radiation. Radiat. Res. 74: 349–362, 1978.

14. Paufler, S. K. and Foote, R. H.: Effect of triethylenemelamine (TEM) and cadmium chloride on spermatogenesis in rabbits. J. Reprod. Fertil. 19: 309–319, 1969.

15. Swierstra, E. E. and Foote, R. H.: Cytology and kinetics of spermatogenesis in the rabbit. J. Reprod. Fertil. 5: 309–322, 1963.

16. Clermont, Y.: Kinetics of spermatogenesis in mammals: seminiferous epithelial cycles and spermatogonial renewal. Physiol. Rev. 52: 198–236, 1972.

17. Berndtson, W. E.: Methods for quantifying mammalian spermatogenesis: a review. J. Anim. Sci. 44: 818–833, 1977.

18. Meistrich, M. L., Reid, B. O. and Barcellona, W. J.: Changes in sperm nuclei during spermiogenesis and epididymal maturation. Exp. Cell. Res. 99: 72–78, 1976.

19. Jackson, H.: Comparative effects of some antispermatogenic chemicals. In: The Regulation of Mammalian Reproduction, S. Segel, R. Crozier, P. A. Corfman, and P. D. Condliffe, Eds., Charles C. Thomas: Springfield, Illinois; pp. 257–270, 1973.

20. Oakberg, C. F.: Gamma-ray sansitivity of spermatogonia of the mouse. J. Exp. Zool. 134: 343–356, 1957.

21. Parvinen, L. M., Soderstrom, K. O. and Parvinen, M.: Early effects of vinblastine and vincristine on the rat spermatogenesis: analyses by a new transillumination-phase contrast microscopic method. Exp. Pathol. 15(2): 85–96, 1978.

22. Homm, R. E., Rustians, C. and Hahn, D. W.: Antispermatogenic effects of 5-Thio-D-glucose in male rats. Biol. Reprod. 17(5): 697–700, 1977.

23. Steinberger, E. and Sud, B. N.: Specific effect of fluoroacetamide on spermiogenesis. Biol. Reprod. 2: 369–375, 1970.

24. Lu, C. C. and Meistrich, M. L.: Cytotoxic effects of chemotherapeutic drugs on mouse testis cells. Cancer Res. 39: 3575–3582, 1979.

25. Withers, H. R., Hunter, N. M., Barkley, H. T. and Reid, B. O.: Radiation survival and regeneration characteristics of spermatogenic stem cells of mouse testis. Radiat. Res. 57(1): 88–103, 1974.

26. Courot, M.: Some results obtained in the irradiation with X-rays of testes of lambs. In: Effects of Ionizing Radiation on the Reproductive System, W. Carlson and F. Gassner, Eds., Pergammon Press: New York: pp. 279–286, 1964.

27. Berndtson, W. E.: Methods for quantifying mammalian spermatogenesis: a review. J. Anim. Sci. 44: 818–833, 1977.

28. Steinberger, E. and Tjioe, D. Y.: A method for quantitative analysis of human seminiferous epithelium. Fertil. Steril. 19: 960–970, 1968.

29. Harasymowycz, J., Ball, L. and Seidel, G. E., Jr.: Evaluation of bovine spermatozoal morphologic features after staining or fixation. Am. J. Vet. Res. 37: 1053–1057, 1976.

30. Holtz, W. and Foote, R. H.: Composition of rabbit semen and the origin of several constituents. Biol. Reprod. 18: 286–292, 1978.

31. Amann, R. P.: Use of animal models for detecting specific alterations in reproduction. Appl. Fund. Toxicol.; in press, 1982.

32. Boucher, J. H., Foote, R. H. and Kirk, R. W.: The evaluation of semen quality in the dog and the effects of frequency of ejaculation upon semen quality, libido, and depletion of sperm reserves. Cornell Vet. 48(1): 67–86, 1958.

33. Amann, R. P.: Effect of ejaculation frequency and breed on semen characteristics and sperm output of rabbits. J. Reprod. Fertil. 11: 291–293, 1966.

34. Freund, M.: Effect of frequency of emission on semen output and an estimate of daily sperm production in man. J. Reprod. Fertil. 6: 269–286, 1963.

35. Desjardins, C., Kirton, K. T. and Hafs, H. D.: Sperm output of rabbits at various ejaculation frequencies and their use in the design of experiments. J. Reprod. Fertil. 15: 27–32, 1968.

36. Amann, R. P., Kavanaugh, J. F., Griel, L. C., Jr. and Voglmayr, T. K.: Sperm production of Holstein bulls determined from testicular spermatid reserves, after cannulation of rete testis or vas deferens, and by daily ejaculation. J. Dairy Sci. 57: 93–99, 1974.

37. Katz, D. F. and Overstreet, J. W.: Sperm motility assessment by video-micrography. Fertil. Steril. 35(2): 188–193, 1981.

38. Overstreet, J. W., Katz, D. F., Hanson, F. W. and Fonseca, J. R.: A simple, inexpensive method for objective assessment of human sperm movement characteristics. Fertil. Steril. 31: 162–172, 1979.

39. O'Connor, M. T., Amann, R. P. and Saacke, R. G.: Comparisons of computer evaluations of spermatozoal motility with standard laboratory tests and their use for predicting fertility. J. Anim. Sci.; in press, 1981.

40. Seidel, G. E., Jr. and Foote, R. H.: Variance components of semen criteria from bulls ejaculated frequently and their use in experimental design. J. Dairy Sci. 56: 399–405, 1973.

41. MacLeod, J. and Gold, R. Z.: The male factor in fertility and infertility. II. Spermatozoan counts in 1000 men of known fertility and in 1000 cases of infertile marriage. J. Urol. 66: 436–449, 1951.

42. Freund, M.: Standards for the rating of human sperm morphology. Int. J. Fertil. 11: 97–180, 1966.

43. Belsey, M. A., Eliasson, R., Gallegos, A. J., Moghissi, K. S., Paulsen, C. A. and Prasad, M. R. N.: Laboratory Manual for the Examination of Human

Semen and Semen-Cervical Mucus Interaction, Press Concern: Singapore; 43 pp., 1980.

44. Eliasson, R.: Analyses of semen. In: Progress in Infertility, S. J. Behrman and R. W. Kistnes, Eds., Little Brown and Co.: Boston; pp. 691–713, 1975.

45. Hammerstedt, R. H.: Monitoring the metabolic rate of germ cells and sperm. In: Reproductive Processes and Contraception, K. W. McKerns, Ed., Plenum Publishing: New York; pp. 353–391, 1981.

46. Thorell, J. I. and Larson, S. M.: Radioimmunoassay and Related Techniques. C. V. Mosby Co.: St. Louis; 1978.

47. Gomes, W. R.: Chemical agents affecting testicular function and male fertility. In: The Testis, Vol. 3, A. Johnson, W. Gomes, and N. Van Demark, Eds., Academic Press, Inc.: New York; pp. 483–554, 1970.

48. Jouannet, P., Czyglik, F., David, G., Mayaux, M. J., Spira, A., Moscato, M. L. and Schwartz, D.: Study of a group of 484 fertile men. I. Distribution of semen characteristics. Inter. J. Androl. 4: 440–449, 1981.

49. Schwartz, D., Mayaux, M. J., Spira, A., Moscato, M. L., Jouannet, P., Czyglik, F. and David, G.: Study of a group of 484 fertile men. II. Relation between age (20–50) and semen characteristics. Inter. J. Androl. 4: 450–456, 1981.

50. Heuchel, E., Schwartz, D. and Price, W.: Within-subject variability and the importance of abstinence period for sperm count, semen volume, and pre-freeze and post-thaw motility. Andrologia 13: 479–485, 1981.

51. Rogers, B. J., Van Campen, H., Veno, M., Lambert, H., Bronson, R. and Hale, R.: Relationship between morphology and human-sperm fertilizing ability. Fertil. Steril. 32: 664–670, 1979.

52. Snyder, P. J., Lipschultz, L. I. and Greenberg, S. H.: In: The Testis of Normal and Infertile Men, P. Troen and H. Nankin, Eds., Raven Press: New York; 539 pp., 1977.

53. Yanagimachi, R., Lopata, A., Odom, C. B., Bronson, R. A., Malin, C. A. and Nicolson, G. L.: Retention of biologic characteristics of zona pellucida in highly concentrated salt solution—use of salt-stored eggs for assessing the fertilizing-capacity of spermatozoa. Fertil. Steril. 31(5): 562–574, 1979.

54. Yanagimachi, R., Yanagimachi, H. and Rogers, B. J.: Use of zona-free animal ova as a test-system for assessment of fertilizing-capacity of human spermatozoa. Biol. Reprod. 15(4): 471–476, 1976.

55. Blazak, W. F., Overstreet, J. W., Katz, D. F. and Hanson, F. W.: A competitive *in vitro* assay of human sperm fertilizing ability utilizing contrasting fluorescent sperm markers. J. Androl; in press, 1982.

56. Federal Register: Proposed guidelines for mutagenicity risks assessments. RP FRL 1563-2. 45(221): 74984–74988, 1980.

57. Kapp, R. W., Jr.: Detection of aneuploidy in human sperm. Environ. Health Perspect. 31: 27–31, 1979.

58. Beatty, R. A.: F-bodies as Y-chromosome markers in mature sperm heads: a quantitative approach. Cytogenet. Cell. Genet. 18: 33–49, 1977.

59. Roberts, A. M. and Goodall, H.: Y-chromosome visibility in quinacrine-stained human spermatozoa. Nature 262: 493–494, 1976.
60. Kapp, R. W., Jr. and Jacobson, C. B.: Analysis of human spermatozoa for Y chromosomal nondisjunction. Teratogen. Carcinogen. Mutagen. 1: 193–211, 1980.

II. GLOSSARY OF TERMS USED IN MALE REPRODUCTION

androgen—a class of steroid hormones produced in the gonads and adrenal cortex that regulate masculine sexual characteristics; a generic term for agents that encourage the development of or prevent changes in male sex characteristics.

backward motility—the movement of a sperm in a reverse direction (toward the middle piece) rather than a forward direction. Note: backward motility is typically caused by a 180° reflection of the middle piece, which may be a secondary abnormality or may be an artifact induced by temperature shock or osmotic shock.

cellular association or **stage**—one of a series of characteristic cellular groupings of different types of germ cells found in a specific area of a seminiferous tubule. Each association contains several layers of germ cells, each layer representing one cell generation. These groupings are not random. Thus, each association contains specific germ cell types in certain developmental phases. For example, spermatogonia of a specific type are always found with primary spermatocytes of a certain developmental phase and spermatids of a certain developmental phase. One cellular association or stage is found at any moment in a given site within a tubule. Cellular associations are a consequence of the synchronous evolution of the different germ cell generations.

circular motility—a clearly discernible motion at a moderate-to-high velocity, but in circles rather than a more or less linear direction.

cohort of germ cells—all germ cells that are the progency of one A-spermatogonium. Since cytokinesis is incomplete, all germ cells in the cohort remain joined by intercellular bridges and develop synchronously.

cycle of the seminiferous epithelium—the complete series of cellular associations occurring in the seminiferous epithelium (6 stages in man; 14 stages in the rat; and generally classified into 8 stages in the rabbit).

daily spermatozoal output—the total number of sperm ejaculated over an interval of at least 7 days after depletion of epididymal reserves, expressed on a per-day basis. Note: for males ejaculating once every 1 to 3 days, after the reserves of spermatozoa in the cauda epididymidis and ductus deferens have been stabilized, daily spermatozoal output will approach daily spermatozoal production.

daily spermatozoal production—the total number of sperm produced per day by the two testes.

duration of spermatogenesis—the interval between the time a stem spermatogonium becomes committed to produce a cohort of spermatids and the release of the resulting spermatozoa from the germinal epithelium. It is likely that the duration of spermatogenesis requires between 4.3 and 4.7 cycles of the seminiferous epithelium (exact values for most species are unknown). It is difficult to establish the time interval between formation of the stem spermatogonium and formation of preleptotene primary spermatocytes, but this interval may equal the duration of between 1.2 and 1.7 cycles of the seminiferous epithelium in many species. Therefore, the term amputated spermatogenesis is occasionally used to refer to the portion extending from formation of the preleptotene spermatocytes through spermiation; this process typically requires about three cycles of the seminiferous epithelium. The entire duration of spermatogenesis would total 4.2 to 4.7 cycles of the seminiferous epithelium (about 72 days in the human and fewer in most animals).

duration of the cycle of the seminiferous epithelium—the interval required for a cell to pass through one complete series of cellular associations. This duration is constant for a strain or species (12.9 days for Wistar rat, 10.7 days for rabbit, and 16.0 days for human). The cycle length is unaffected by environment, hormonal levels, or cytotoxic damage to the germ cells.

efficiency of spermatozoal production—the number of sperm produced per day per gram of testicular parenchyma.

ejaculate—the total seminal sample obtained during ejaculation.

ejaculation—the expulsion of semen through the urethra.

emission—deposition of sperm and fluids from the caudae epididymidis and ductuli deferentia and fluids from the accessory sex glands into the pelvic urethra.

flagellating spermatozoon—a sperm (not stuck to the glass slide) whose position does not change, although its tail moves back and forth.

follicle-stimulating hormone or **FSH**—a glycoprotein hormone secreted by the anterior pituitary of vertebrates that promotes spermatogenesis and stimulates growth and secretion of the Graafian follicle.

luteinizing hormone or **LH**—glycoprotein hormone secreted by the adenohypophysis of vertebrates that stimulates hormone production by interstitial cells of gonads.

maximum tolerated dose (MTD)—the highest dose that can be given during a chronic study without a possibility of shortening an animal's life other than through its carcinogenicity.

meiosis—two divisions of primary spermatocytes to first form secondary spermatocytes and secondly to form spermatids. Cells are called primary or secondary spermatocytes.

nonmotile spermatozoon—a sperm that does not quiver or move a discernible distance during visual observation.

percentage of motile sperm—the percentage of sperm that are progressively motile, circularly motile, or backward motile; conventionally estimated as a subjective observation of sperm in a diluted sample of semen viewed with a phase-contrast microscope. Note: this percentage can be determined objectively using one of several procedures.

percentage of progressively motile sperm—the percentage of sperm that are progressively motile (excluding circularly motile and backward motile sperm); conventionally estimated as a subjective observation of sperm in a diluted sample of semen viewed with a phase-contrast microscope. Note: this percentage can be determined objectively using one of several procedures.

primary abnormality—an abnormality of sperm morphology originating during spermatogenesis, often associated with the head. Fertilization of an ovum by the spermatozoon characterized by a primary abnormality is unlikely.

progressive motility—a clearly discernible, fairly continuous, forward motion at a moderate-to-high velocity in a reasonably linear path. Progressive motility is greater than 25 μm/sec for human sperm. Note: in nonfrozen semen, many sperm will rotate on their long axis while swimming progressively, although in frozen-thawed semen, progressive motility may not be accompanied by cellular rotation. Also, the composition of the buffer used to dilute a sample of semen can influence whether a motile sperm will rotate or swim without rotation (flat). Rotation about the long axis and the helical beat of the tail often move the head of the sperm in a zig-zag path rather than a true linear path.

quantitative evaluation or **objective evaluation**—an analytical measurement of sperm motility or velocity performed by a nonbiased instrument rather than visually by an individual.

quivering spermatozoon—a sperm that rotates slightly on its long axis or oscillates; characteristic of some sperm recovered from the efferent ducts or rete testis.

secondary abnormality—an abnormality of sperm morphology induced during epididymal transit or ejaculation, usually associated with the tail. When a secondary abnormality is induced in a spermatozoon, its competitive ability to fertilize an ovum is reduced.

semen—a mixture of sperm and fluids from the excurrent ducts and accessory sex glands.

seminal volume—the volume of an ejaculate (expressed in milliliters).

seminiferous epithelium—the normal cellular components within the seminiferous tubule consisting of Sertoli cells and germ cells (spermatogonia, primary spermatocytes, secondary spermatocytes, and spermatids). Sertoli cells are somatic cells that are usually nondividing in adult animals and probably are important for metabolic exchange between the germ cells in the luminal compartment and that, by means of Sertoli-Sertoli junctions, form the blood-testis barrier. They also aid in coordination of spermatogenesis and have an endocrine function.

spermatogenesis—the sum of the transformations that result in formation of spermatozoa from spermatogonia and continued formation of a fairly constant number of uncommitted spermatogonia. The entire spermatogenic process is initiated in early embryonic development and continues after birth and puberty as a consequence of continual renewal of stem cells. At birth two cell types are found within the seminiferous tubule: supporting cells, which give rise to the Sertoli cells of the puberal male, and the gonocytes, which will develop into spermatogonia. The intense proliferation of germ cells and the subsequent release of spermatozoa do not occur randomly. Rather the germinal elements always follow the same pattern of development (unless particular cells and their progeny degenerate) within males of a species.

spermatozoal velocity—the velocity with which a progressively motile or circularly motile sperm moves. Spermatozoal velocity is conventionally expressed on a subjective scale from 0 (low velocity) to 4 (maximum velocity) but should be expressed as μm/sec on the basis of quantitative measurements.

spermiation—release of spermatozoa from the germinal epithelium into the lumen of the seminiferous tubule. Prior to release the germ cells are called spermatids, and after spermiation they are called spermatozoa.

spermiogenesis—the differentiation of spermatids from spherical cells with considerable cytoplasm to characteristically shaped cells with a highly condensed nucleus and scant cytoplasm but with a flagellum. Cells are called spermatids. Based on changes in the spermatid acrosome, spermiogenesis can be considered as a continuum consisting of four phases: Golgi, cap, acrosome, and maturation. In addition to acrosomal evolution, condensation of the nuclear material and formation of the flagellum occur.

subjective evaluation—a visual estimate subject to observer bias and error.

testosterone—a biologically potent androgenic steroid that may be released from the gonads and adrenal glands.

total spermatozoa per ejaculate—the total number of spermatozoa in an ejaculate (determined as the product of seminal volume times spermatozoal concentration and expressed as 10^6). Note: the total number of sperm per ejaculate, not spermatozoal concentration, provides the best information on the number of spermatozoa produced by the testes, since spermatozoal concentration is influenced by the relative contributions of the accessory sex glands diluting the bolus(es) of sperm transported during emission from the ductus deferens and cauda epididymidis.

twitching spermatozoon—a sperm that occasionally or continuously moves a short distance with a violent motion and then comes to rest, at least momentarily, before an additional twitch or jump. The twitch or jump need not be in a forward direction.

CHAPTER 4

CURRENT STATUS OF, AND CONSIDERATIONS FOR, ESTIMATION OF RISK TO THE HUMAN CONCEPTUS FROM ENVIRONMENTAL CHEMICALS

E. Marshall Johnson
Jefferson Medical College, Thomas Jefferson University
Philadelphia, PA 19107

Definition and Scope

Teratology is the study of the causes, mechanisms, and sequelae of perturbed developmental events in species of animals that undergo ontogenesis. This report is restricted to a consideration of factors influencing the current status of risk assessment of teratologic effects of environmental agents. It is considered a preliminary document touching upon the major considerations basic to quantitative estimation of risk to development of the conceptus following exposure of pregnant animals to environmental agents. This document provides no definitive means for assessing risks to the human conceptus, since no documented or validated system for such assessment has yet been established. Basic to risk estimation is hazard assessment, which requires quantification and validation of reliable end point assays. This document briefly discusses the factors and scientific considerations upon which degrees of confidence applicable to contemporary studies of teratology are to be based. Some additional considerations in evaluating experimental data (e.g., acute versus chronic exposures) have not been covered explicitly, but references are provided to aid the reader in gathering further information.

Impact of Developmental Abnormalities on Humans

Approximately 50% of human conceptuses fail to reach term, and perhaps as many as half of those lost are structurally abnormal (1). Approximately 3% of newborn children are found to have one or more significant congenital malformations at birth, and by the end of the first postnatal year, approximately 3% more (2, 3) are found to have developmental malformations. An additional group, whose size is difficult to estimate, has functional abnormalities of the nervous, respiratory, gastrointestinal, immunologic, and other systems. Some unknown proportion of these abnormalities may be due to environmental insult during prenatal life.

Causes of Congenital Malformations

Relatively little is known about the specific causes of most human congenital defects. It is estimated that 10 to 15% of all human congenital malformations are due to environmental agents and another 10 to 15% to hereditary factors (i.e., gene mutations and chromosomal aberrations). The remainder are considered to result from unknown causes and from complex interactions between multifactorially determined hereditary susceptibilities and micro-environmental factors precipitating abnormal developmental sequences within the conceptus and its associated membranes. To date, only a relatively small number of specific environmental agents and factors have been identified as causing human malformations (4).

From the above, it is concluded that although regulatory controls on man-made environmental agents may reduce the incidence of developmental abnormalities, they will not totally prevent them. It must be recognized that indications from animal experiments of adverse effects of environmental agents on development may not always be corroborated by observations of perturbed development in human populations. Nevertheless, and in full recognition of these qualifiers, standard animal testing is presently considered the best available method for predicting risk of congenital malformation in human beings prior to human exposure. Information derived from such testing can be used to detect and to estimate the magnitude of hazard posed by specific substances to human prenatal development and can serve as a basis for estimation of risk.

Qualitative Evaluation of Risk Potential

Interspecies comparisons

Inherent interspecies differences complicate extrapolation of animal test results to direct determination of human risk. Because a species identical to the human in all relevant characteristics does not exist, interspecies differences between human beings and the test species must be considered when data are being evaluated. Interpretation of these inherent interspecies differences is complicated by species differences in metabolism and pharmacokinetics of the test agent and in developmental and other attributes characteristic of the species. Very little is currently understood about the extent and nature of the interplay among these many factors as they may affect the production of a teratogenic event.

Since human beings are manifestly heterogeneous, there is little doubt that human populations will contain broad degrees of susceptibility and resistance to the possible adverse prenatal effects of environmental agents. Because this heterogeneity is largely determined by genetic variability, it has been reasoned that stocks of animals bred at random are the most appropriate models for testing teratogenicity. However, in order to estimate the degrees of susceptibility that may exist within human populations, both the average response of the test group and the extent of responses within it must be considered. This goal can be achieved to some extent by using several stocks of animals. To make such a procedure even more sensitive and useful, several inbred strains may also be tested, since this procedure increases the likelihood that a range of sensitivities will be uncovered (5). For instance, genetically controlled variations in embryonic face formation account partly for the sensitivity of certain mouse strains to spontaneous (6) and teratogen-induced (7, 8) cleft lip and isolated cleft palate.

Dosing and mode of administration

The test agent should be administered over a range of doses, including a level sufficient to produce signs of maternal toxicity in the particular species used. If a teratogenic response is observed, a dose-response relationship should be determined for the agent and that specific teratogenic effect. In using test animals, the selection of dosing intervals must take into account the varying degrees of sensitivity during organogenesis in that species, the possibility of enzyme induction or other modifying processes that could result from repeated administration of the test material, and the practical aspects of administration that would make the dosing comparable to that which would likely occur with human exposure.

The route of administration of the test agent may significantly affect the outcome of an experiment. In general, the route of exposure for test animals should mimic that of human exposure where possible, although valuable data may be obtained from other routes of exposure as well. Differences in the response of a species to the route, dose, and vehicle used for exposure to the test agent may result in significant variations in blood and tissue levels of the agent in the maternal and embryo-fetal units (9). These factors may or may not be of direct significance to teratogenesis, but they must be recognized as being potentially significant.

Placental transfer

The anatomy and physiology of the placentas of experimental animals and man present a diverse spectrum of maternal-fetal connections (10). The chorioallantoic placenta of the human is approximated by that in some non-human primates, whereas the common experimental animals have, in addition, a yolk sac placenta, which also structurally and functionally joins embryo and mother. The extent to which the yolk sac may supplement or complement transfer of a previously untested chemical via the chorioallantoic circulation is largely unpredictable. In most of these species (e.g., rat, mouse, rabbit, guinea pig), the yolk sac placenta may play a major role in maternal-fetal exchange of substances during early organogenesis. The chorioallantoic placenta, which is readily available for convenient study at term, is in most cases a totally different structure from that effecting transfer during the critical stages of development; therefore great care must be exercised to avoid unwarranted extrapolation from studies of term chorioallantoic placenta to presumptions for the function of the two placental structures present earlier in gestation. Lipid solubility, ionic charge, molecular size, and specific structural configuration all appear to contribute to the transfer of chemicals between mother and fetus. Little or no relationship may exist between the embryonic and fetal concentration of agents and their possible teratologic effect, since potent teratogens do not always accumulate in the fetus at concentrations greater than those of agents with low teratogenic potential. Consequently, increased concentration ratios between the conceptus and mother do not necessarily allow predictability of teratogenic or other embryotoxic potential (11, 12). Little is currently known about the sites of action of teratogenic agents; therefore, any component of the entire maternal-placental—embryo-fetal unit and all combinations of such should be considered as possible site(s) for teratogenic action, until the mechanism of teratogenic action for given agents is better understood.

Pharmacokinetics and metabolism

Other variables that may affect the teratogenicity of an agent in various species include pharmacokinetics and metabolism and those exogenous factors that may affect these parameters. Some of the factors to be considered when evaluating data from these experiments are seasonal and circadian effects on development and metabolism (13, 14); interaction of pharmacokinetic and placental hemodynamics (15); possible sites of action of agents; sites of maternal, placental, and embryonic-fetal metabolism; and deposition and/or depression or induction of metabolic enzymes (9, 16). Certain agents may stimulate or inhibit enzyme systems, such as liver microsomal enzyme systems. In some cases single doses at critical periods in gestation induce a greater teratologic response than divided doses on several consecutive days (17–21). Maternal and embryo-fetal nutritional and endocrine states in various species may interact with and/or alter metabolism and pharmacokinetics (22), as may species-specific effects resulting from repeated administration of the test agent, saturation of metabolizing enzymes, and inhibition or induction of biotransforming enzymes (16, 23).

Basic to interpreting data from studies of teratology is documentation of a dose-response relationship and determination of a treatment level below which adverse effects are not evident in the data available (no-observed-effect level or NOEL). Threshold levels may be encountered, and dose levels can exist below which development of the conceptus suffers no observable deleterious effect at term. The no-observed-effect level does not guarantee absolute safety, because uncertainty may result from biological and/or statistical variation. Failure to detect a deleterious effect on the end point examined could indicate the absence of a deleterious effect, but absence of observed effect also could occur if the magnitude of an effect were below the limit of statistical detection ability.

Mechanisms of action

The mechanisms underlying abnormal embryonic development are not well understood. It has proven difficult to determine whether an observed incidence of abnormal development is the result of an agent or one of its products acting directly on the conceptus or its placenta, or if it is achieved indirectly through an initial effect on the mother. Therefore, the primary site of action by an agent capable of disrupting development may or may not be the specific malformed organ and may not even be within the conceptus. Whether or not a chemical is evenly distributed within the mother and conceptus, its action on a particular tissue or organ may be dependent on cellular interactions and the particular developmental events characteristic of specific ontogenetic stages. Increased knowledge of these ontogenetic events and the interaction of toxic agents or their products with them is needed both to understand the resulting defects and to enable better extrapolation of effects seen in one species to predictions of potential effects in another.

Animal Studies

Standard teratogenicity testing

Schardein (24) has discussed in some detail the current methodology and testing approach initially outlined in the 1966 Food and Drug Administration's (FDA's) guidelines for reproductive studies and in the 1967 and 1978 World Health Organization's recommendations, which are further specified in the U.S. Environmental Protection Agency's proposed guidelines. Numerous countries have required studies that are generally similar but that vary in particulars. The object of the standard protocols is to expose animals to test materials before breeding of the parental generation, during *in utero* development and lactation, and in some instances into adult life of the offspring. To achieve their goals, the experiments are designed in three phases or segments, with a multigeneration test for reproductive effects required in some instances.

The first phase, or Segment-I protocol, calls for dosing of both male and female animals to begin some calculated time prior to breeding. Treatment of the young males begins 60 days prior to breeding, and exposure of the females to the test substance begins two weeks prior to breeding. Dosing continues for both sexes during the breeding interval and for the impregnated females throughout pregnancy and lactation. Other major details of the Segment-I protocol could be described here, but these will be slighted to emphasize the basics.

The Segment-I protocol is supposed to examine for possible adverse effects on estrus; sexual performance; formation of the gametes; their release from the gonad, transport, and interaction to form a zygote; and zygote passage to and implantation into the decidua. Because dosing of the dam continues after mating, the protocol could reveal effects on placental formation and its function; and because dosing continues throughout gestation and lactation, the protocol could reveal adverse effects on embryonic or fetal development and on delivery, nurture, and postnatal development of the pups. Adverse effects of the test material on the supportive functional parameters essential for normal occurrence of each of the above could also become evident. These effects could be as diverse as effects on food intake or altered endocrine status. This study is usually made in rats, and by indicating problem areas, it can serve as a preliminary to later studies.

The second protocol is oriented more specifically to detect effects on embryonic development. The study is usually made in both rats and rabbits. The Segment-II study requires that the males not be treated with the test compound and that treatment of the pregnant females not begin until after decidual implantation of the blastocysts has occurred. Treatment ceases at the end of major organogenesis, usually considered as the time of closure of the secondary palate in the species. Autopsy is performed the day before expected delivery, when the term fetuses are collected for gross external examination, after which they are examined for skeletal development and internal soft-tissue morphology.

The goal of this experiment is to detect adverse effects of a test material on the developmental events characteristic of major organogenesis in the embryo.

A Segment-III evaluation is a perinatal and postnatal study requiring treatment of the dams only. The test agent is administered during the last third of pregnancy and throughout lactation. Treatment is not scheduled to begin until after the period of major embryonic development is completed.

The Segment-III safety evaluation was designed to detect adverse effects of substances on fetal development as well as those developmental processes that continue into infancy and adolescence. It is in this study that potential effects on postnatal behavior of the young are usually evaluated.

A rather elaborate multigeneration protocol is employed for evaluating selected substances for effects on reproduction over three generations. The goal of the multigeneration protocol is to reveal effects caused by accumulated toxicity or by agents effective at low concentration. These protocols for safety evaluation have had detailed discussion (14, 25), and for each a data base of considerable size has accumulated. They are not considered as final, however, because there is a need for flexibility and exercise of scientific judgment (26), which could improve their detecting ability in some instances. There is also some justification for their revision in light of research findings in related fields since their inception.

There are four types of developmental defects: gross anatomical, death in utero, growth retardation, and functional deficit (4). Currently, the first three of these end points are the only ones that have a data base sufficient to ensure confidence in their applicability for use in regulatory decisions. Functional status has been studied broadly only in recent years and soon may develop end point assays with specific applicability.

Examination of fetuses to identify gross anatomical defects often entails judgmental and subjective appraisals based on criteria or standards established by individual laboratories. The routine test as performed by many laboratories applying FDA's Good Laboratory Practices requires highly trained technical and professional personnel. Even though general standards for defining the limits of normality and associated terminology have not been established, in general when selected compounds have been evaluated by various laboratories, similar findings have been demonstrated by those using the routine teratology test and its methods for examining the young (27, 28).

The overwhelming majority of chemicals known to be teratogenic in human beings have been demonstrated to be teratogenic in one or more common laboratory species. Many other agents shown to be teratogenic in laboratory animals have not yet been documented as teratogens in humans. The difference may be due to insufficient epidemiologic data, dissimilarities of exposure levels, or differences in end points analyzed. A teratogenic response in one species or strain should be considered indicative of a potential teratogenic hazard for human beings. However, negative responses in a few species of experimental animals do not necessarily guarantee absence of adverse effects in human conceptuses. In the routine teratology test, no one species has been consistently more predictive of human teratogenicity than another species.

Functional teratogenicity testing

Functional alterations may prove to be sensitive indicators of teratogenic potential. Among those that have been studied following prenatal exposure, a broad and complex range of behavioral effects has been described. There is concern that these effects may occur at doses below those producing gross structural defects or prenatal death (29). Current literature is based largely on studies of rodents, particularly rats, in which it has been demonstrated that exposure to chemicals during periods from early organogenesis through pubescence can result in behavioral impairments. To detect such effects more efficiently, reliable and sensitive test procedures are being developed in several laboratories (30, 31). Although there are no agreed-upon testing methods, current studies routinely include the end points in the following areas: (a) reflex ontogeny, (b) habitation and reactivity, (c) learning and problem solving, (d) activity level, (e) motor skills, and (f) sensory processes.

Other functional parameters demonstrated to be affected by prenatal exposure to chemicals include fertility; reproduction; the endocrine system; immune competence; xenobiotic metabolism; and various physiologic parameters, including cardiovascular, renal, gastrointestinal, respiratory, and hepatic functions (32). Finally, late sequelae of prenatal exposure to chemicals may be manifested postnatally as cancers or shortened life span (33, 34).

Gross structural defects or significant growth retardation may complicate analysis of data from tests of function, and alertness to potential confounding factors is essential. Permanent changes in functional systems should be viewed as indicating the potential for an adverse effect in human beings. Transient changes or delays in functional ontogeny are still not understood, and their significance must be further evaluated.

Short-Term Testing Procedures

Prioritizing of chemicals for in-depth study

As a prelude to estimation of potential risks, a series of biological and informational factors may be applied to a new substance to possibly trigger further testing to some level in a tier system of evaluations for teratologic effects. It is considered highly desirable that substances be prioritized for testing to focus research attention more readily on substances injuring conceptuses at doses significantly below those toxic to adults. In attempting to list the factors to be taken into consideration, the need for short-term systems became evident because of the large number of evaluations needed and the fact that many of the available data would be in category 2 below. Listed below are the factors that, when applicable, would make a substance a high-priority candidate for further testing. Within each of the two categories, the factors are listed in decreasing order of importance.

1. Biological effects data possibly available regarding a substance: Suspected human teratogenicity; Teratogenicity in domestic

animals or wildlife established; Short-term teratology test indicating a significant developmental hazard potential; Adult toxic dose/developmental toxic dose ratio large; Toxicity documented in the adult at low dosage;
2. Additional information available regarding a substance: Large numbers of women exposed; Bioaccumulation evident; Persistence of substance in environment; New substance; Involuntary exposure.

The number of agents in use and potentially impinging on human development is already vast and is increasing rapidly. Some unknown small fraction of these may be potentially harmful to human conceptuses at doses below those obviously deleterious to adults. Short-duration and low-cost methods for detecting and prioritizing those substances posing the greatest potential hazard to the conceptus are needed. Because standard tests in animals are quite costly, only a rather small number of substances of potential teratogenic risk can be evaluated each year. This situation requires development and validation of short-term methods that will permit rapid and meaningful testing of these chemicals. It is necessary to develop, validate, and use assays that will permit more economical testing of a larger number of agents than could be tested rapidly and conveniently by standard teratogenicity evaluations. Validation should consist of various forms of positive correlation between the results of such tests and those found in conventional *in vivo* test procedures. Particular attention should be directed to correlations with known human teratogenic responses whenever reliable data are available. Included should be chemicals already known to have significant hazard potential for the conceptus, as well as chemicals considered as lacking such potential. If properly validated short-term tests were to indicate either potential hazard or safety, such determinations would be helpful for establishing a priority system for further tests aimed toward quantitative risk assessment.

Characteristics of short-term assays

Short-term tests might be considered as either preliminaries to more detailed evaluations, or they might serve as efficient means to detect those substances capable of posing the greatest hazard to the conceptus. Whether they serve either or both of these slightly different goals, the tests should possess certain attributes: they should be rapid, economical, and reproducible from one laboratory to another; should have easily identifiable end points; and ideally should prioritize substances according to their potential for posing hazards to the conceptus. Confidence in their applicability would be increased by demonstration of dose-response relationships. They should give minimal false negatives; it is understood that false positives can be explored further in more elaborate animal testing. Ideally, the system should encompass as many as possible of the developmental events known to occur in the conceptus.

Short-term tests may serve as preliminary screens to aid in the detection of possibly teratogenic hazards. To accomplish this, several such tests would probably have to be performed concurrently or sequentially. It must be remembered that such indications of teratogenic hazard potential must be used prudently for estimating risk to human beings. Risk estimation can only be achieved by the use of systems that have been extensively validated, and to date, only the more routine standard testing methods are considered applicable to this use.

Potential short-term systems

In vivo. Two *in vivo* systems have been advanced as possible short-term systems. One is an abbreviated version of a standard teratology test protocol using the maternal maximum tolerated dose and neonatal evaluation shortly after birth (35). The second is evaluation of homeotic shifts that may prove effective for detecting minimal expression of teratogenic hazard potential (36). Each system has potential merit, but as in the *in vitro* systems, needs careful peer review or detailed validation.

In vitro. Artificial invertebrate "embryos," embryonic insect cells, amphibian and fish embryos, or organs of avian and mammalian embryos (palatal shelves, tooth bud, kidney mesenchyme, pancreas, bone primordia, lens, sex organs, etc.) have the potential to serve as the basis for *in vitro* systems. Table 12 lists a number of potential *in vitro* systems. In these procedures, cells, organs, or whole embryos have been exposed to various chemicals and their effects measured with the end point permitted by each system. When attempted in a few instances, adequate dose-response relationships were obtained by some systems. In their present state, the systems listed in Table 12 have been only partially validated (36–50), and their closer examination is necessary.

TABLE 12   Some *In Vitro* Short-Term Systems
Currently in Various Stages of Development

	System	Developmental parameters monitored	References
Invertebrates	Hydra	Various	36
	Planaria	Regeneration, dose-response relationship of developmental toxicity	37, 38
	Drosophila cells	Differentiation	39
Fish	Zebra fish	Dose-response relationship of developmental toxicity	40
Vertebrate cell culture	Chick embryo neural crest	Morphology, differentiation	41
	Chick embryo limb bud mesenchyme	Differentiation	41
	Mouse tumor cells	Cell attachment	42
	Teratocarcinoma stem cells	Differentiation (*in vivo* or *in vitro*)	43
Organ culture	Mouse embryo limb bud	Growth, dysmorphogenesis, differentiation	44, 45 46, 47
Whole embryo culture	Rat, mouse, chick	Growth, dysmorphogenesis, histogenesis	16, 48 49, 50

Quantitative Risk Assessment

Quantitative risk assessment is based on the relationship between laboratory findings and expected human response. If an agent demonstrates teratogenicity in any mammalian species, some concern about prenatal human exposure to the agent is justified. The level of concern is to be tempered by numerous considerations, not the least of which is the extent of maternal toxicity evident at the dose level needed to elicit a toxic response in the conceptus (51). It is assumed that margins of safety applied to the experimental data in test species can be used to estimate an allowable exposure in pregnant women. It is considered that no-observable-effect and/or threshold levels of exposure do exist (52) for at least some teratogens. The determination of human risk requires the definition of moderating (or modulating) conditions such as the distribution of the compound within the environment; its pattern of use and exposure (whether intermittent or chronic); and the identification of those subpopulations that may be at high risk as a result of factors such as life style, age, occupation, etc.

The use of animal test systems under highly controlled experimental conditions has conditional validity for defining human risk. Although only warning systems at best, laboratory experiments can provide, in addition to the factors already mentioned, two types of information that may be useful for estimation of the potential human risk. These are (a) the ratio of the adult and developmental toxic doses and (b) the shape of the curve of the teratogenic dose response. Although not markedly informative to date, more detailed delineation of projected effects may be obtained through use of pharmacokinetic information, focusing on access of the agent to relevant site(s) of teratogenic action (53). However, knowledge of teratogenic mechanisms and identification of the sites actually relevant must be obtained before these considerations can achieve their full potential utility.

It is often necessary to conduct animal experiments at dosage levels exceeding estimated levels of human exposure to increase the likelihood that a weak teratogen will produce an apparent effect and to compensate for the relatively small numbers of animals used in the test. This requires extrapolation of results from experimental dosage levels to lower levels of human exposure. There is no uniform basis for selecting the appropriate mathematical model for such extrapolation.

Safety factors may be applied to establish acceptable dosage levels that are expected to yield acceptable levels of risk. The size of the safety factor depends upon the quality and quantity of the biological effects data available.

For many biological systems, the dose-response curve tends to flatten at low doses, and for some teratogens this is an important consideration (54). Hence, decreasing dosage by a safety factor of F will generally decrease risk by more than a factor of F. That is, if the upper confidence limit on the risk is U at an experimental dosage of d, the potential risk at a lower dosage of d/F is predicted to be less than U/F for the test animal. The uniformity with which this would apply to potential teratogenic hazards is undetermined as is the degree of interspecies uniformity for the difference between the adult (A) toxic and developmental (D) toxic doses. Presence or absence of uniformity in the A/D ratio or slope of the dose-response between studies in different species would also influence the magnitude of safety factors.

Priorities for Future Research in Teratology

The areas of research in teratology recommended below focus on two broad objectives: (a) development of practical and informative testing systems with which to evaluate both the plethora of chemicals now in existence and those yet to be developed and (b) scientific advancement in teratology so that the currently employed and largely standard test systems can become more useful and reliable for human risk estimation. The second objective does not imply that currently available methods cannot be used for human risk estimation. An opposite view is held, and within limits, such estimations are possible at the present time on the basis of data from current state-of-the-art studies. It is felt, however, that methods are needed to identify more rapidly those chemicals potentially the most hazardous and to expand the understanding and applicability of all test methods.

1. The degree to which the end point determinations of adverse effects on development encountered in the standard protocols predict adverse effects in other species (especially humans) has not been reported in detail sufficient for precise quantification of human risk. Such studies are encouraged as are those that may indicate how the predictive ability of tests in animals can more precisely herald human responses.

2. Validated methods are needed for rapid and inexpensive detection of substances uniquely toxic to conceptuses (i.e., substances that are embryotoxic at doses below those producing adult toxicity).

3. A better understanding of mechanisms of teratogenic action or elucidation of the steps in the pathway between exposure and effect might significantly improve and refine end point assays. Similar studies of pathogenesis are needed for effects on biochemical and physiological systems in the dam, uterus, and placenta.

4. Development of a broader data base on comparative metabolism and pharmacokinetics correlated with teratologic end points may eventually enhance ability to make interspecies extrapolations.

5. There is a need to develop and validate methods to detect and quantify possible functional impairments.

6. Methods are needed to detect and predict additive or synergistic effects more effectively.

REFERENCES

1. Hertig, A. T.: The overall problem in man. In: Comparative Aspects of Reproductive Failure, K. Benirschke, Ed., Springer-Verlag: New York; pp. 11–41, 1967.
2. McKeown, T. and Record, R. C.: Malformations in a population observed for five years after birth. In: Ciba Foundation Symposium on Congenital Malformations, G. E. W. Welstenholme and C. M. O'Conner, Eds., Little Brown: Boston; pp. 2–16, 1963.
3. Mellon, G. W. and Kalzenstein, M.: Increased incidence of malformations – chance or change? J. Am. Med. Assoc. 187: 570–573, 1964.
4. Wilson, J. G.: Environment and Birth Defects. Academic Press: New York; 305 pp., 1973.
5. Kalter, H.: Interplay of intrinsic and extrinsic factors. In: Teratology: Principles and Procedures, J. G. Wilson and J. Warkany, Eds., University of Chicago Press: Chicago; pp. 57–80, 1965.
6. Trasler, D. G.: Pathogenesis of cleft lip and its relation to embryonic face shape in A/J and C57BL mice. Teratology 1: 33–49, 1968.
7. Trasler, D. G.: Aspirin-induced cleft lip and other malformations in mice. Lancet 1: 606–607, 1965.
8. Trasler, D. G. and Fraser, F. C.: Time-position relationships with particular reference to cleft lip and cleft palate. In: Handbook of Teratology, Vol. 2, J. G. Wilson and F. C. Fraser, Eds., Plenum Press: New York; pp. 271–292, 1977.
9. Larsson, K. S.: Contributions of teratology to fetal pharmacology. In: Fetal Pharmacology, L. O. Boreus, Ed., Raven Press: New York; pp. 401–418, 1973.
10. Beck, F.: Comparative placental morphology and function. Environ. Health Perspect. 18: 5–12, 1976.
11. Waddell, W. J. and Marlowe, G. C.: Disposition of drugs in the fetus. In: Perinatal Pharmacology and Therapeutics, B. L. Mirkin, Ed., Academic Press: New York; pp. 119–268, 1976.
12. Wilson, J. G., Scott, W. J., Ritter, E. J. and Fradkin, R.: Comparative distribution and embryotoxicity of methotrexate in pregnant rats and rhesus monkeys. Teratology 19: 71–80, 1979.
13. Barr, M., Jr.: Prenatal growth of Wistar rats: circadian periodicity of fetal growth late in gestation. Teratology 7: 283–288, 1973.
14. Layton, W. M.: An analysis of teratogenic testing procedures. In: Congenital Defects, New Directions in Research, D. T. Janerich, R. G. Skalko and I. H. Porter, Eds., Academic Press: New York; pp. 205–217, 1974.
15. Wolkowski-Tyl, R. M.: Strain and tissue differences in cadmium-binding protein in cadmium-treated mice. In: Developmental Toxicology of Energy-related Pollutants, D. D. Mahlum, M. R. Sikov, P. L. Hackett and F. D. Andrew, Eds., Technical Information Center: Oak Ridge, Tennessee; pp. 568–585, 1978.

16. Fantel, A. G., Greenaway, J. C., Juchau, M. R. and Shepard, T. H.: Teratogenic bioactivation of cyclophosphamide *in vitro*. Life Sci. 25: 67–72, 1979.
17. Russell, L. B., Badgett, S. K. and Saylors, C. L.: Comparison of the effects of acute, continuous, and fractionated irradiation during embryonic development. Int. J. Radia. Biol., Suppl: 343–359, 1960.
18. Wilson, J. G.: Effects of acute and chronic treatment with Actinomycin D on pregnancy and the fetus in the rat. Harper Hosp. Bull. 24: 109–118, 1966.
19. King, C. T. G., Horigan, E. and Wilk, A. K.: Fetal outcome from prolonged versus acute drug administration in the pregnant rat. In: Drugs and Fetal Development, M. A. Klingberg, A. A. Abramovici and J. Chemke, Eds., Plenum Press: New York; pp. 61–75, 1972.
20. Tuchmann-Duplessis, H.: Teratogenic Action of Drugs. Pergammon Press: New York; 1965.
21. Belisle, R. J. and Long, S. Y.: Tolbutamide treatment of pregnant mice: repeated administration reduces fetal lethality. Teratology 13: 65–70, 1976.
22. Neubert, D., Merker, H.-J., Kohler, E., Krowke, R. and Barrach, H. J.: Biochemical aspects of teratology. In: Advances in the Biosciences, G. Raspe, Ed., Pergammon Press: Oxford; pp. 575–622, 1971.
23. Bakay, B. and Nyhan, W. L.: Effects of Thalidomide and Chlorcyclizine on the biosynthesis of nucleic acids and proteins in fetal and maternal tissue of the rat. J. Pharmacol. Exp. Ther. 171(1): 109–117, 1970.
24. Schardein, J. L.: Drugs as Teratogens. CRC Press: Cleveland; pp. 9–12, 1976.
25. Kelsey, F. O.: Present guidelines for teratogenicity studies in experimental animals. In: Congenital Defects, New Directions in Research, D. T. Janerich, R. G. Skalko and I. H. Porter, Eds., Academic Press: New York; pp. 195–204, 1974.
26. Golberg, L. M. B.: Discussion pp. 53–55. In: Methods for Detection of Environmental Agents that Produce Congenital Defects, T. H. Shepard, J. R. Miller, and M. Marois, Eds., North-Holland Publishing Co.: Amsterdam; 1975.
27. Wilson, J. G.: Methods for administering agents and detecting malformations in experimental animals. In: Teratology: Principles and Techniques, J. G. Wilson and J. Warkany, Eds., University of Chicago Press: Chicago; pp. 262–277, 1965.
28. Staples, R. E. and Schnell, V. L.: Refinement in rapid clearing technique in the KOH-alizarin-red-S method for fetal bone. Stain Technol. 39: 61–63, 1963.
29. Hutchings, D. E.: Behavioral teratology: embryopathic and behavioral effects of drugs during pregnancy. In: Studies on the Development of Behavior and the Nervous System, Vol. 4, Early Influences, G. Gottlieb, Ed., Academic Press: New York; pp. 7–34, 1978.

30. Vorhees, C. V., Brunner, R. L. and Butcher, R. E.: Psychotropic drugs as behavioral teratogens. Science 205: 1220–1225, 1979.
31. Buelke-Sam, J. and Kimmel, C. A.: Development and standardization of screening methods for behavioral teratology. Teratology 20: 17–29, 1979.
32. Kimmel, C. A.: A profile of developmental toxicity. In: Developmental Toxicology, C. A. Kimmel and J. Buelke-Sam, Eds., Raven Press; in press, 1981.
33. Rice, J. M.: Perinatal period and pregnancy: intervals of high risk for chemical carcinogens. Environ. Health Perspect. 29: 23–27, 1979.
34. Spyker, J. M.: Assessing the impact of low-level chemicals on development: behavioral and latent effects. Fed. Proc. Fed. Am. Soc. Exp. Biol. 34: 1835–1844, 1975.
35. Chernoff, N. and Kavlock, R. J.: A potential *in vivo* screen for the determination of teratogenic effects in mammals. Teratology 21: 33A–34A, 1980.
36. Johnson, E. M.: A subvertebrate system for rapid determination of potential teratogenic hazards. J. Environ. Pathol. Toxicol. 4: 153–156, 1980.
37. Best, J. B., Morita, M., Ragin, J. and Best, J., Jr.: Acute toxic responses of the freshwater planarian, *Dugesia dorotocephala,* to methyl-mercury. Bull. Environ. Contam. Toxicol.; in press, 1981.
38. Best, J. B., Morita, M. and Abbotts, B.: Acute toxic responses of the freshwater planarian, *Dugesia dorotocephala,* to chlordane. Bull. Environ. Contam. Toxicol.; in press, 1981.
39. Bournias-Vardiabasis, N., Terplitz, R. L. and Seecof, R. L.: An *in vitro* assay for teratogenesis. Teratology 21: 29A, 1980.
40. Streisinger, G.: Invited discussion on the possible use of zebra fish for the screening of teratogens. In: Methods for Detection of Environmental Agents that Produce Congenital Defects, T. H. Shepard, J. R. Miller and M. Marois, Eds., North-Holland Publishing Co.: Amsterdam; pp. 59–61, 1975.
41. Wilk, A. L., Greenberg, J. H., Horigan, E. A., Pratt, R. M. and Martin, G. R.: Detection of teratogenic compounds using differentiating embryonic cells in culture. *In Vitro* 16: 269–276, 1980.
42. Braun, A. G., Emerson, D. J. and Nichinson, B. B.: Teratogenic drugs inhibit tumor cell attachment to lectin-coated surfaces. Nature 282: 507–509, 1979.
43. Filler, R.: An *in vitro/in vivo* coupled prescreen to identify teratogens requiring metabolic activation. Teratology 21: 37A, 1980.
44. Kochhar, D. M.: The use of *in vitro* procedures in teratology. Teratology 11: 273–288, 1975.
45. Neubert, D. and Barrach, H. J.: Significance of *in vitro* techniques for the evaluation of embryotoxic effects. In: Methods in Prenatal Toxicology: Evaluation of Embryotoxic Effects in Experimental Animals, D. Neubert, H. J. Merker and T. E. Kwasigroch, Eds., Georg Thieme: Stuttgart; pp. 202–209, 1977.

46. Manson, J. M. and Simons, C. R.: *In vitro* metabolism of cyclophosphamide in limb bud culture. Teratology 19: 149–158, 1977.
47. Kochhar, D. M. and Agnish, N. D.: Teratogenic testing *in vitro*. In: Toxicity Testing *In Vitro,* R. M. Nardone, Ed., Academic Press: New York; in press, 1981.
48. New, D. A. T.: Techniques for assessment of teratologic effects: embryo culture. Environ. Health Perspect. 18: 105–110, 1976.
49. Brown, N. A., Goulding, E. H. and Fabro, S.: Ethanol embryotoxicity: direct effects on mammalian embryos *in vitro*. Science 206: 573–575, 1979.
50. Klein, N. W., Vogler, M. A., Chatot, C. L. and Pierro, L. J.: The use of cultured rat embryos to evaluate the teratogenic activity of serum: cadmium and cyclophosphamide. Teratology 21: 199–208, 1980.
51. Johnson, E. M.: Screening for teratogenic potential: are we asking the proper question? Teratology 21: 259, 1980.
52. Staples, R. L.: Teratogens and the Delaney Clause. Science 185: 813, 1974.
53. Young, J. F. and Holson, J. F.: Utility of pharmacokinetics in designing toxicological protocols and improving interspecies extrapolation. J. Environ. Pathol. Toxicol. 2: 169–186, 1978.
54. Jusko, W. J.: Pharmacodynamic principles in chemical teratology: dose-effect relationship. J. Pharmacol. Exp. Ther. 183: 469–480, 1972.

CHAPTER 5

OTHER CONSIDERATIONS:

EPIDEMIOLOGY, PHARMACOKINETICS,

AND SEXUAL BEHAVIOR

Robert W. Goy, *University of Wisconsin, Madison, WI 53706*
Kenneth B. Bischoff, *University of Delaware, Newark, DE 19711*
Carol J. Hogue, *University of Arkansas, Little Rock, AR 72201*
Lynn Rosenberg, *Boston University Medical Center, Cambridge, MA 02138*

Epidemiology: Methods and Limitations

Epidemiology has been defined as the study of the distribution and determinants of disease and injury in humans. It focuses on the occurrence of disease in groups of individuals or populations rather than in any single individual (1). Ideally, reproductive and teratologic effects of environmental agents would be assessed in epidemiologic studies of human populations because of the difficulties inherent in extrapolating from other species. However, ethical considerations render randomized controlled trials generally unfeasible. If one cannot experiment, then one can only observe, but in some circumstances even observation is not possible (e.g., risk assessment of new chemicals before they are introduced into the human environment).

Observational epidemiologic studies can be classified into those that generate hypotheses and those that formally test hypotheses and quantify risks. The following list is not an exhaustive delineation of all possible epidemiologic approaches in these categories, but it includes those which may be most useful for environmental risk assessment.

Hypothesis—generating studies

Case reports are a source for raising suspicions about substances that might be teratogens or reproductive hazards (e.g., an astute clinician's association of thalidomide with phocomelia). However, only very striking or very rare outcomes can be detected in this manner and often after a considerable length of time. For the vast majority of pregnancy outcomes, formal epidemiologic studies involving appropriate comparison groups are required.

Correlational studies evaluate the patterns of morbidity or mortality in populations where classification is made on the basis of aggregates of individuals as distinct from single individuals (e.g., geographic-specific spontaneous abortion rates correlated with area-specific air pollution levels).

In *demographic studies,* routinely collected information is used to estimate disease rates in populations composed of individuals classified by limited demographic characteristics (e.g., age and sex), allowing for the identification of subgroups at particularly high risk and of changes in the rates over time.

Population-based registries can detect changes in the incidence of the outcomes being registered (e.g., spontaneous abortions, low birth weight, birth defects, neonatal deaths). If placed in selected areas of suspected high risk and "clean" areas of presumed low risk, they may point up differences potentially resulting from environmental causes. Their case materials are a useful resource for mounting case-control studies of suspected environmental hazards (see below).

**Analytic studies for formally testing hypotheses and
     quantifying risks**

In the *case-control* design, a series of individuals with an observed effect (the outcome of interest) and a series of unaffected individuals are compared with respect to their previous exposure to the environmental agent of interest. The case-control method is most appropriate for the study of extremely rare outcomes, such as ambiguous genitalia and specific birth defects, and relatively rare outcomes, such as infertility and ectopic pregnancy. It is not useful for the study of very rare exposure unless the study is conducted in a selected setting with sufficiently large numbers of exposed persons (e.g., occupational settings). Case-control studies are not feasible when previous exposures cannot be ascertained.

In *cohort studies,* cohorts of exposed and unexposed individuals are followed for the subsequent occurrence of the outcomes of interest. This design may be the most desirable method for studying fairly common outcomes (e.g., spontaneous abortions), for determining conception rates, and for evaluating subtle indications of reduced fertility, such as variations in interpregnancy interval.

Limitations

All observational studies are subject to certain limitations. Studies classified as hypothesis-generating lack information on potential distorting factors; for this reason, among others, they cannot be used to establish cause-effect relationships. Formal analytic studies do have this capacity if they are valid (i.e., relatively free of biases attributable to selection, measurement, and confounding).

If losses to follow-up are related to outcome status (cohort studies) or if entry into the study is related to exposure status (case-control studies), then *selection bias* will be present. This can occur in industrial settings, for example, if individuals who are exposed to hazardous substances tend to leave the industry and become lost to follow-up because they become ill.

Errors in measurement of exposure or outcome, if unequal between the groups being compared, can lead to overestimation or underestimation of an effect. Equal measurement errors will always lead to attenuation of an effect, and this is a particular problem when exposure or outcome is difficult to measure, as is the case with many environmental exposures and some reproductive outcomes. In cohort studies, there is particular concern that the ascertainment of subsequent outcome be unbiased, while in case-control studies, there is particular concern that the measurement of prior exposure to the agent of interest be unbiased.

Because observational epidemiologic studies deal with non-randomized populations, a central concern is whether the groups being compared are similar in all relevant characteristics. If they differ in factors related to both the exposure and the outcome, then *confounding bias* will be present. Properly conducted epidemiologic studies will make allowance for all known risk factors of the health outcome of interest, either in the design or in the analysis.

For assessment of the validity of a particular study, detailed information about recruitment and participation of the study population, measurement of the parameters of interest, method of analysis, and efforts to assess potential biases must be available. A single epidemiologic study, even if valid, can seldom by itself rule out chance or bias as the explanation of an observed association. Establishment of causal associations usually requires the accumulation of consistent evidence from valid studies of human populations. That cause precedes effect must also be demonstrated. Belief in a particular hypothesis can be strengthened by evidence from animal studies, by a biologically plausible mechanism, and by a dose-response relationship. In general, the stronger an association, the easier it is to establish a causal association. Conversely, the smaller the effect, the more difficult it is to demonstrate. Failure to detect an effect may simply reflect inadequate sample size or insufficient time for the outcome to become manifest.

This brief review touches on only a few of the potential limitations of observational epidemiologic studies. The assessment of the validity of any particular study requires extensive knowledge of epidemiologic methods and experience with their application.

Possible data sources and useful approaches

Currently few epidemiologic studies attempt to detect human teratogenic and reproductive hazards or to quantify their effects. Furthermore, there is no systematic application of epidemiologic methods for this purpose. It would be desirable to have programs specifically designed to raise suspicions and to test hypotheses. To be effective, these programs must be supported on an ongoing basis.

Before pilot testing any new epidemiologic program, however, the potential usefulness of existing studies and data bases should first be evaluated. Several examples of potentially useful systems are given below.

There are several registries of birth defects in the United States, for example, the Birth Defects Monitoring Program of the Center of Disease Control, which collects information from selected hospitals throughout the country, and the birth defects registries of metropolitan Atlanta and of Nebraska and Florida. The development in selected regions of population-based registries of reproductive health outcomes (including birth defects, ectopic pregnancies, and spontaneous abortions) could point to potential environmental hazards. Even in a particular geographic area, clusters of cases or changes in rates over time could suggest a source of environmental contamination.

Vital statistics have been analyzed from time to time, depending upon the interest of the investigator. For example, infant mortality rates have correlated with chlorination levels of public water supplies in New York (1). In addition, vital statistics have been used as indicators of reduced male fertility in an occupational setting (2, 3). A systematic ongoing analysis of vital statistics data in relation to routinely collected environmental data might be quite useful for raising suspicions about environmental hazards.

Two ongoing surveillance systems based on the case-control approach are currently in operation: one is designed to discover and to evaluate adverse drug effects that are serious enough to warrant hospitalization (4, 5), and the second is directed to the discovery and evaluation of drug teratogenic effects (6). In principle this methodology is applicable to the discovery of environmental agents that are reproductive hazards or teratogens. For the surveillance of occupational exposures, programs could be located in specified areas of the country where occupational exposures to suspected hazards are high. The application of this methodology to the study of nonoccupational environmental exposures is more difficult, in part because individuals may not be aware of what they have been exposed to.

The cohort method has been used to identify several health hazards in occupational cohorts (7, 8). Other cohorts that might be useful are enrollees in health maintenance organizations (HMOs) (see, for example, Ref. 9). However, an HMO data base has the limitation that only outcomes that come to medical attention can be studied. Moreover, no HMO currently has a computerized data base in a form that would be useful for the conduct of epidemiologic studies of environmental exposures. A large investment would be required to build and maintain such a data base.

Pharmacokinetics

Pharmacokinetics can be defined as the quantitative study of the absorption, disposition, metabolism, and elimination of drugs, poisons, and other chemical agents in the body. It is important to evaluate pharmacokinetic variables at different doses and routes of exposure to understand the toxicological significance of exposure.

Pharmacokinetics can be employed for at least two purposes: definition of the concentration levels of the agent in blood or in tissues where the site of action is presumably located, and quantitative description and prediction of the relevant concentration levels, usually with a mathematical model. The first should be routinely done to the extent possible as an aid in interpreting other measurements being made. The second requires much more comprehensive study but has the potential for predictive purposes such as risk assessment.

At this time, there are several basic textbooks of pharmacokinetics: Notari (10) presents an elementary overview, but with many applications; Wagner (11) and Gibaldi and Perrier (12) provide collections of the basic mathematical models and solutions with illustrations of their use. These classical treatments permit organization of pharmacokinetic data, along with some biological interpretations of amounts of an agent in the "central" regions of the body (blood, vital organs) versus "peripheral" regions (other tissues). However, for use of measured levels in specific tissues, models incorporating what is known about quantitative aspects of anatomy and physiology have been found useful (13, 14). Another important feature of this alternative approach is to enable use of known physiological and pharmacological differences between animal species to define some of the critical parameters for quantitative extrapolation to man. A review is given by Dedrick (15), and suggestions for defining similarities between animal species are described by Dedrick and Bischoff (16).

A survey of application of the above pharmacokinetic approaches to some areas of toxicology is given by Gehring et al. (17), and further discussions are in chapters of World Health Organization Environmental Health Criteria (18) and Filov et al. (19). Some specific issues of importance concerning reproductive and teratogenic effects are described by Young and Holson (20).

When pharmacokinetics is applied to the specific area of teratology, the major determinants of the teratogenic agent's reaching and accumulating in the conceptus are the usual aspects of pharmacokinetics in the mother, plus the unique features of transplacental transport, and pharmacokinetics in the conceptus. The maternal pharmacokinetics may be monitored by the blood half-life (20), although it may also be desirable to have more complete details of the disposition into the uterine tissue, as well as the presence of active metabolites and inducible catabolic enzymes, later mobilization of stored agent, and any differences between pharmacokinetics in chronic versus acute exposures. The uptake and disposition into the conceptus may be partially predicted from knowledge of placental membrane transport parameters (models of oxygen and glucose transport may be a useful basis [22]), specific and nonspecific binding, and other features of the developing fetus. It is crucial to determine these effects during the period of major organogenesis.

Few available studies have applied pharmacokinetic principles to specific areas of female or male reproductive organs, especially with reference to formulating models that could be used for predictive purposes. In one of the few, uptake of cancer chemotherapeutic agents into the human uterus has been successfully described by a physiological pharmacokinetic model, which was then used to formulate clinical dosage regimens (22). In another, Lee and Dixon (23) present the results of their innovative study of the pharmacokinetic determinants of uptake into male gonads.

Clearly, much more needs to be done before pharmacokinetics can be routinely utilized as an adjunct in better defining the basis for risk assessment of reproductive and teratogenic toxic effects. However, information obtained using the reasonably well developed methods described in the earlier references should aid in developing methods to resolve some of the issues.

Sexual Behavior

Introduction

Overview. The behavioral aspects of reproduction encompass a broad spectrum of activities including courtship behavior, sexual behavior, parental behavior, and a variety of social activities that subtly influence the probability of reproductive success. The scope of this discussion is limited primarily to sexual behavior for the following reasons.

- This behavioral aspect of reproduction has received the most detailed and extensive attention from clinicians and laboratory investigators.
- Evaluation procedures for sexual behavior of a variety of animal species are well established.
- Choices can be made among several existing standardized procedures currently in use in laboratories around the country.
- Observational methods are simple and direct, and workers at a moderate level of skill can be quickly trained to obtain reliable measurements.
- Many of the testing procedures recommended in the following presentation can provide insight into the probable locus of action of the putative toxicant, and this could not be as easily achieved if the scope of the investigations was extended to include at this time other behavioral aspects of reproduction.

The presentation that follows attempts to establish the impact and causes of sexual dysfunction in humans, to discuss methods of assessing human sexual behavior, and to indicate the difficulties associated with investigations of human sexuality when there are neither controls nor standard norms. The evaluation of sexual behavior patterns in animals are presented as simple tallies of specific motor responses; however, it will be emphasized that many elements of human sexual behavior are unique, having no animal counterpart, thus making uncertain any extrapolation of data on animal sexual behavior to humans.

Definition and scope.   The study of sexual behavior encompasses the measurement of normal and abnormal function as well as the identification of the factor(s) responsible for the impairment of sexual behavior. The quantitative measurement of sexual functioning involves the establishment of norms or averages for groups and for the individual and most often focuses on coitus itself. For humans more extensive and varied measures are necessarily employed, which include sexual imagery, sexual fantasy, varieties of overt sexual experience, self concept and gender identity, assessment of interpersonal relationships, choice of sexual object, and level of sexual skill.

For the most part, animal models available today do not provide data that might be required for assessing human sexual functioning and for identifying the factors responsible for imparied expression of sexual behavior. Nevertheless, important advances made in the study of animal sexual behavior provide at least for the initial screening of toxicants that could deleteriously affect human sexual conduct. To identify the factors responsible for normal and impaired sexual behavior, investigators of animal sexual behavior have identified three separate components: sexual attractiveness, sexual initiative, and sexual responsiveness. The current working assumption is that these factors have a much broader generalizability across species than any isolated species-typical behavioral response or activity (e.g., mounting). The evidence and arguments favoring this working assumption have been set forth persuasively by Beach (24), who uses the alternative terminology of attractivity, proceptivity, and receptivity to designate the three factors. Accepted systems of measurement have been worked out for a variety of laboratory animals including the rat and macaque monkeys (25−27).

It should be realized from the outset that manifest sexual behavior reflects the functional integrity of a broad system comprising elements of drive and reward, perception, sensory function, motor performance, the physicochemical actions of gonadal hormones on neural and somatic tissues, and, finally, central nervous system processing and coordinating of the interactions of all of these elements. An efficient screening system utilized for detection of toxic effects should attempt at some stage to distinguish between general motoric disability (ataxia) and impairment of specific sexual reflexes; between general lassitude and loss of specific sexual interest or motivation; and between the impaired production of gonadal hormones and the impaired actions of these hormones. At this time, however, no simple and efficient test of sexual behavior or tests designed to measure sexual attractiveness, initiative, and responsiveness automatically determine whether elements of the broad system are impaired either as a result of general debilitation or selectively and specifically with regard to sexual performance. Currently available tests, while not permitting decisions about the specificity of the effect of a toxic substance, can serve as early warning signals that normal reproductive function has been impaired.

Impact of sexual dysfunction on humans.   Data on the incidence of human sexual dysfunction and its spontaneous remission are neither extensive nor very reliable. Certainly the most common clinical problems are primary and secondary anorgasmia in females and *ejaculatio praecox* and erectile impotence in males. These disorders, however, represent extremes of dysfunction that are unacceptable to most humans, and those so affected commonly seek clinical help. Less extreme forms of inadequate sexual response clearly exist and are often tolerated, but only in the sense that professional counseling is not sought. Even though many individuals are reluctant to seek professional help, the importance of sexual behavior and sexual gratification to the overall quality of life and individual well-being is generally recognized. Many individuals are willing to relinquish reproductive capabilities (through vasectomy or other contraceptive means) to enjoy fewer restrictions on sexual activity. Few people, however, will relinquish sexual gratification to gain contraception.

The importance attached to sexual gratification by individuals in our society implies that sexual inadequacy, even when tolerated, may not be without serious consequences. Our monogamous social system depends in a very fundamental way upon a sexual contract between two individuals. Failure to achieve, or even reduction of, sexual satisfaction seriously threatens the interpersonal relationship, as the growing number of marriage counselors recognize. How much of the growing sexual and marital discord is attributable to sociopsychological factors and how much might be attributable to disturbances in the physiological systems underlying sexual performance is not known. The possibility exists, however, for toxic substances in the environment to cause disturbances in sexual performance and thereby contribute to interpersonal discord.

Causes of impaired sexual performance. Sexual dysfunction in human beings is poorly understood. Many sexual disorders are primarily psychogenic and respond well to psychological treatment. Others that are resistant to psychological approaches seem to originate in specific genetic factors, early experience, or a combination of genetic and experiential determinants.

Endocrinopathies, especially abnormalities of the gonadal hormones, have marked influences on the pattern of sexual behavior displayed by animals, and although their influence is less well described for humans, it cannot be said that their role is negligible. For both the male and the female, inadequate gonadal hormone activity commonly results in deficient sexual performance. Subnormal effectiveness of gonadal hormones can be due to (a) deficiencies in production, (b) deficiencies in bioavailability, and (c) deficiencies in target organ sensitivity and/or responsiveness.

Androgen deficiency affects male behavior in two distinct ways. First, during early stages of development (probably before birth in humans) deficiencies in androgen lead to incomplete development of central neural and peripheral somatic structures essential for the expression of masculinity and male behaviors including, but not limited to, male sexual behavior. Second, during adolescence and adulthood, deficiencies in androgen are associated with reduced sexual responsiveness and sexual initiative.

Behavioral disorders associated with excessive androgen have not been identified for the male, although there are recurrent suggestions that excessive amounts during early stages of development lead to permanent androgen insensitivity. In the female, however, excessive androgen during early developmental stages leads to the development of masculine behavioral and somatic characteristics and, in some species, to the suppression or loss of feminine behavior traits. This suppression of feminine traits can include sexual behavior, and female sexual responsiveness can be only reduced. In adulthood, excessive androgen in female humans may lead to measurable somatic virilization (such as hirsutism and clitoromegaly) without any marked effect on psychological and behavioral traits. Increases in sexual initiative and responsiveness may be large enough to be distressing and disruptive to an established interpersonal relationship. In nonhuman primates, androgens have also been implicated in the control of proceptivity (sexual initiative), but not in the control of receptivity. In other mammalian animals, excessive androgen in adulthood may cause a sharp increase in the frequency of malelike mounting activity and aggression with or without concomitant alterations in female sexual behavior. Most of the psychological and somatic changes induced by excessive androgen in adulthood are partially or totally reversible when the hormonal excess is eliminated; however, some of the more dramatic somatic changes (e.g., voice changes and hirsutism) are irreversible.

Estrogen and progestagens play essential but incompletely understood roles in the regulation of female sexual response. These hormones are produced and secreted in much larger amounts by the ovaries than by the testes or the adrenals in normal physiological conditions. Whereas human female sexual behavior does not depend entirely upon the actions of estrogens and progestagens, its expression is greatly facilitated by their actions on both central and peripheral neural and somatic tissues. In animals, especially the common laboratory forms, the ovarian hormones are much more essential to the expression of female sexual behavior than in human beings. Generally, the effective estrogen is estradiol and the effective progestagen is progesterone. These two steroid hormones act synergistically in the induction of both proceptivity and receptivity in rats, mice, hamsters, and guinea pigs. The two hormones may also act antagonistically, however, and which relationship obtains depends upon whether or not the estrogen has been free to act for a specifiable period of time without any concurrent actions of a progestagen. The synergistic relationship depends upon the sequential action of an estrogen followed (usually 36 to 48 hours later) by the action of a progestagen. An antagonistic relationship will be evidenced whenever a progestagen and an estrogen are both present throughout the period of observation or study.

Excessive estrogenization acts to lengthen the period or duration of receptivity and proceptivity. An established norm of eight hours for the duration of receptivity in a colony of rats can be extended to 12 or 14 hours by excessive estrogenization. In extreme cases, excessive estrogenization can extend receptivity indefinitely.

Excessive progesterone has no measurable effect if the period of stimulation is brief. If the period of excessive stimulation is protracted, however, receptivity and proceptivity can be indefinitely suppressed or inhibited. The antagonistic effect of progestagens is transitory and reversible when these hormones are brought back to physiologic concentrations.

It is difficult but not impossible to distinguish between the antagonistic effects of excessive progestagen and a deficiency in estrogenization. A deficiency of estrogen, like excessive progestagenization, has the primary characteristic of weak or absent female sexual response. A distinction between the two possible causes of impaired sexual response can be made by institution of appropriate experimental hormone administration to ovariectomized females.

Excessive estrogen or progestagen during early periods of development can produce permanent deficiencies in female sexual response in a variety of laboratory animals. Comparable data for human beings do not exist.

Sequelae of estrogen and/or progestagen excess or deficiency in males have not been well worked out. Supraphysiologic levels of estrogen have been administered to human males in cases of prostatic cancer. Sexual drive and erectile potency sometimes decline in these cases, presumably because the estrogens block the release by the pituitary of testis-stimulating hormone, and an androgen deficiency results. Similar effects could be obtained in some laboratory animals (the guinea pig), but not in others (the rat, in which excessive estrogens mimic androgens in the potentiation of male sexual activity).

The effects of hormone excess and deficiency could occur when chemical substances mimic or antagonize physiological actions of the relevant gonadal hormone. Other chemical agents could enhance the degradation of steroidal hormones in the liver or kidneys and thereby reduce or limit their effectiveness. Still other chemicals could either act on the hypothalamic-pituitary system to modify the release of trophic substances essential for the normal production of the gonadal hormones or act directly upon the glandular tissues responsible for their production.

Many factors, aside from alteration of or interference with hormonal support, can act to impair sexual behavior. These factors are difficult to assess in standard laboratory tests, either because no suitable animal model can be found or because appropriate assessment would involve procedures too elaborate and costly for routinization. Although testing for alteration or interference with the hormonal support of sexual behavior assesses only a limited aspect of requirements for human sexual adequacy, it has the advantage that the information gained is reliable, quantitative, and amenable to use in estimating the risk to human sexuality posed by specific chemical substances.

Qualitative evaluation of risk potential

Interspecies comparisons. Requirements for genetic variability in the test model animal that approximates that encountered in the human population have already been discussed in the section titled "Interspecies Comparisons" in Chapter 4. Highly inbred strains ought to be generally avoided unless several are used to determine the range of sensitivity to the test substance.

Known and suspected differences among species in the manner in which gonadal hormones regulate sexual behavior mandate the use of more than one species. For example, the major androgen produced by the testis is testosterone in most mammals. This hormone is metabolized within somatic and neural cells to a variety of other steroids including estradiol and dihydrotestosterone. In some species, like the rat, the estradiol derived from bioconversion of testosterone is a potent stimulator of male sexual behavior in the adult and a potent masculinizer of the developing brain in the fetus and neonate. In contrast, in the guinea pig this estrogen metabolite of testosterone is without any measurable stimulating effect on male sexual behavior when it is given to castrated adults. The view is widely held that the display of male sexual behavior depends upon the intracellular conversion of testosterone to estradiol in the normal male rat, whereas testosterone acts either directly or via conversion to dihydrotestosterone on the neural tissues mediating male sexual behavior in the guinea pig.

The "rat model" for cellular utilization of testosterone (by conversion to an estrogen) is valid for hamsters and some but not all inbred strains of mice. The "guinea pig model" is valid, based on very limited data, for the rhesus monkey and also for humans.

This species difference is important because erroneous conclusions are possible if testing is limited to a single species. Any putative toxicant that blocks intracellular aromatizing enzymes needed for bioconversion of testosterone to estrogen would impair adult male rat sexual behavior, but the same compound would not likely have an effect on sexual behavior of male guinea pigs, rhesus monkeys, or humans.

Other species differences, too numerous to detail here, include differences in the role of specific neural structures, in the contribution of specific neurotransmitters, in the amount and kind of carrier protein that is present in the bloodstream and binds and transports the steroid hormones, in the chemical structure of the pituitary trophic hormones, and certainly in the form and normal frequency of sexual expression. All of these species differences argue for the use of more than one species in screening for toxicity as well as for judicious choices when only a few are to be used. In short, the choice of a species to use as a model animal places profound and subtle limits on evaluating the toxic consequences of any chemical agent, and these limits have to be reckoned with.

Certain relatively simple and easy-to-conduct tests could serve as a preliminary screen to indicate the degree of likelihood of an agent's affecting either the early sexual differentiation or adult expression of sexual behavior. Based on the assumption that chemical substances that pass the placenta and gain access to the fetal tissues are more likely to affect early development than those that fail to pass through the placenta, a relatively simple and efficient study of the distribution of the radioactively labeled chemical substance could be carried out. It is also reasonable to use radiolabeled material in adult animals to determine whether the substance crosses the blood-brain barrier and has the potential of acting directly on nervous tissue. These simple tests, of course, are not specific indicators that sexual behavior would be altered by the putative toxicant. Positive findings from these tests would merely serve the purpose of indicating increased likelihood.

Other considerations. It is reasonable to assume that a wide variety of other factors are important in facilitating extrapolation of animal tests of a toxicant to the estimation of risk to humans. These include dosages of putative toxicant used, route of administration, duration and frequency of exposure, species thresholds and sensitivities to the chemical substance, and specific pharmacokinetics and pharmacodynamics of the test compound. Whenever information exists for humans on any of these factors, either for the specific test compound or a closely related substance, an effort should be made to select an animal model that most closely parallels the human to increase the applicability of the animal test results.

Despite the advantages of objectivity, ease of administration, reliability, and wealth of background information, tests of animal sexual behavior in the present context have severe limitations. First and foremost is the high degree of uncertainty that results of animal tests could be extrapolated to human sexual behavior. It is likely that extrapolation would be good if a putative toxicant completely blocked the neurological actions of the sex hormones (especially the androgens), since hormonal support for sexual behavior and for the fetal differentiation of sexual and/or sex-related behavior is a factor common to both animals and humans. However, humans and animals differ greatly in the numbers and kinds of nonhormonal factors influencing the expression of sexual behavior. Accordingly, when a putative toxicant acts only on one or a subset of nonhormonal factors, there is a strong likelihood that animal test results will not correspond to effects (or lack thereof) on human sexual expression.

A second area of concern is the nearly total lack of background information on effects of known toxicants on sexual behavior in either animals or humans. This deficiency thwarts any present attempt at formulation of procedures for quantitative risk assessment based on findings from animal tests. This situation can be remedied only by providing encouragement of the appropriate research on animal models as well as intensive studies of humans exposed to known toxic agents.

Animal studies

Evaluation of sexual behavior in adulthood. Observations of sexual behavior in adult animals can be made by easily trained nonexperts. Useful assessments of the status of sexual behavior can be made from simple tallies of the frequency of occurrence of specific motor responses and the latent period from the beginning of a standardized test to the occurrence of the specific response. These are the operational measures of initiation, attractiveness, and responsiveness.

The procedures described in this section are designed to permit reliable, sensitive analyses of the effects of potentially active chemical substances on male sexual behavior. A considerable body of knowledge gathered in the last 60 years reveals that the sexual patterns of rats and guinea pigs can provide such data. Further, the existence of extensive data bases on these two species provides the possibility of a preliminary indication of mechanism of action underlying observed treatment effects, since determinants of various aspects of these complex patterns have received much study. Should more extensive and expensive testing of a chemical be indicated, dogs, nonhuman primates, or other species may be appropriate. Methods described below can be adapted to such species using behavioral testing procedures described by Dewsbury (28) and in the references therein.

In all tests, one sex should be treated so that treatment effects may be detected uncomplicated by effects of the agent's acting on the opposite sex. Where the probability of a treatment effect is quite low, it may be more economical to combine procedures for male and female treatments into a single protocol. However, the risk that three rather than two studies may be required if such procedures are used should be recognized.

Assessing sexual behavioral patterns of males. Effects of various toxicants can be evaluated as they alter the normal complex behavioral patterns of male rats and guinea pigs. There are some considerable advantages to toxicological inquiry in studying the behavior of male animals that have been castrated and given physiological hormone replacement and exogenous testosterone. This procedure obviates the possibility that impaired sexual performance might be due to toxic insult to the hypothalamic-pituitary-testicular axis or to the testis itself. However, inasmuch as castration and replacement therapy are complicated techniques in themselves, testing the intact animal should serve as an adequate preliminary screen.

In studying the normal copulatory behavior of laboratory rats, three classes of events are generally distinguished — mounts, intromissions, and ejaculations. With the first the male mounts the female from behind, displays shallow pelvic thrusting, but neither gains vaginal penetration nor displays the stereotyped pattern of dismounting. Intromissions begin similarly, but the male achieves a single deep thrust and dismounts in a vigorous and stereotypical pattern. Ejaculations occur only after several intromissions and are characterized by an intravaginal thrust that is longer and deeper than that of intromissions. Sperm are transferred only on ejaculations. The male mounts the female during mounts, intromissions, and ejaculations, but the three classes of events are distinguished as just indicated. During pair mating copulatory events occur in "ejaculatory series," with each series terminated by an ejaculation and separated from a resumption of copulation by a postejaculatory refractory period. In standard testing cages, males normally display a mean of approximately seven ejaculatory series before attaining an arbitrary, but standard, satiety criterion of 30 minutes with no intromissions or ejaculations.

Standard measures of male copulatory behavior include mount latency (ML), time from start of a test to the first mount or intromission; intromission latency (IL), time from the start of a test to the first intromission; ejaculation latency (EL), time from the first intromission of a series to its terminal ejaculation; intromission frequency (IF), number of intromissions in a series; mount frequency (MF), number of mounts in a series; mean interintromission interval (MIII), mean interval separating the intromissions within a series; and postejaculatory interval (PEI), time from ejaculation to the next intromission. Male receptivity may be quantified by dividing the number of male chase and follow-bouts by the total number of female approaches (29).

Because various of these measures can be affected selectively, specifically, and in combination, an accurate interpretation of a treatment effect requires a full complement of these measures. As an example, suppose a treatment interfered with the process of penile erection. Males with such problems often mount females at rates much higher than normal as they repeatedly attempt to effect intromission. Without a full complement of measures, such an effect might be mistaken for an *increase* in libido rather than as a deficit. Similarly, a treatment that alters MIII may secondarily affect IF. In addition, with a full set of measures, one can evaluate the control group in relation to animals used in previous studies (see references below) to ensure that it is providing an appropriate baseline for comparison.

Full descriptions of copulatory behavior in male rats can be obtained in Beach and Jordan (30), Dewsbury (27), Larsson (31), and Sachs and Barfield (32).

Copulatory behavior in male guinea pigs differs from that in male rats in several important respects. First, whereas rats display but a single intravaginal thrust on each mount with intromission, guinea pigs display repetitive thrusts on a single insertion. Second, whereas male rats rarely, if ever, ejaculate on the first mount with intromission, such occurrences are more frequent in guinea pigs. Third, although male rats normally display several ejaculations per test session, the occurrence of the first ejaculation generally effectively terminates copulatory activity in guinea pigs. In other respects, the copulatory patterns of male guinea pigs are quite similar to those of male rats. Similar measures can be used.

Descriptions of copulatory behavior in guinea pigs can be found in Young (33) and Young and Grunt (34). Various measures of preliminary aspects of courtship and mating described in these papers may be useful.

Test of copulatory behavior should be conducted during the dark phase of the diurnal cycle. By testing during the second half of the dark phase, behavior generally is more reliable, quicker, and less variable — making for a more efficient and sensitive test (35). Tests should be conducted at approximately the same time on each day.

Males and females should be familiar with the testing arenas via introduction several times on days before test days.

In tests for male behavior, males are generally placed in the arenas for five to ten minutes, after which the female is introduced, effectively beginning the test. Tests may be terminated and scored as negative if there is no copulatory activity within a predetermined time (e.g., 15 minutes).

Tests of guinea pigs should be terminated at the occurrence of ejaculation. Those of rats should be continued for two or three ejaculatory series. Such tests may require an average of 45 minutes in rats. It may be feasible to test several pairs of rats simultaneously in cages close to each other, if the only behavioral patterns to be scored are those discussed above.

For reasons of reliability and predictability, it is recommended that female mating partners be brought into behavioral estrus with exogenous hormones. Female guinea pigs must first be ovariectomized; this may or may not be done with female rats. For either intact female rats or spayed guinea pigs, good results can be obtained with an intramuscular injection of 0.1 mg of estradiol benzoate three days before testing and 1 mg of progesterone approximately six hours before testing. Somewhat lower doses can also be used. Females should be placed briefly with a vigorous, nonexperimental "indicator" male immediately before testing to ensure that the injection regimen has been effective in inducing receptivity. A single female rat in estrus can be used to evaluate sexual performance of at least three males. A single female guinea pig should not be used for more than two males.

There are many factors, both quite specific and highly nonspecific, that can alter copulatory behavior. If there are gross increases or decreases in body weight or activity levels, changes in sexual behavior are probably secondary to more general effects. If body weight and general activity is near normal and copulatory behavior is altered, however, greater specificity of action probably is indicated. Some indication of the nature and degree of effect can be determined by considering the constellation of measures altered, the magnitude of effect, and reversibility. By comparing these changes to those described in the literature as resulting from other treatment, some preliminary indication as to probable mechanism of action can be gained. Any alteration requires some further analysis. Such subsequent studies may be directed at analyzing neural, endocrine, and other systems to determine whether or not the effect seems appreciable and likely to affect humans.

Assessing sexual behavior patterns of females. A substantial and useful background of behavioral data exists for both rats and guinea pigs from a number of inbred strains as well as genetically heterogenous stocks. It is possible to evaluate proceptivity, receptivity, and attractiveness in female rats in a single test paradigm with a stud male and to evaluate receptivity in the female guinea pig.

The intact and normally functioning female rat displays a period of estrus ("heat") that lasts from 6 to 11 hours about every 4 to 5 days. As long as the female is not mated, estrus recurs regularly. Recurrent estrus also occurs in the unmated female guinea pig, but the interval between receptive episodes lasts 14 to 17 days. In both species, sexual behavior depends upon appropriate ovarian secretion of estradiol and progesterone. When the ovaries are removed, sexual behavior is no longer displayed. Proceptive and receptive behaviors are displayed in close temporal proximity and have similar hormonal requirements (36).

The behavioral response indicative of normal receptivity is the lordosis posture assumed by the female during mounting by a male partner. Degree of receptivity is estimated in a quantitative fashion by dividing the number of lordosis responses displayed by the female by the number of times she is mounted by her male partner in a standardized test. This derived measure is called the *receptivity quotient* or, alternatively, the *lordosis quotient.* The measure is more useful in the rat than in the guinea pig, because male rats are normally multiple mounters, whereas male guinea pigs often mount only once during a mating test. For the female guinea pig, therefore, an alternative procedure for quantifying receptivity is often used. The procedure, described fully elsewhere (37, 38), involves manual stimulation of the animal's rump and perineum by the human observer and measurement of the degree or duration of the lordosis response to such stimulation. During mating with a stud male, female attractiveness may be quantified by measuring the latency between introduction of the female and a male approach, follow, and mount (29).

Proceptivity can be measured quantitatively in the female rat by recording the frequency and timing of displays of a variety of motor patterns including female solicitations and approaches to the male partner, darting, hopping, and ear vibration. These proceptive patterns generally are displayed just prior to the occurrence of male mounting responses, but they may occur at any time when the male is quiet or inactive.

Full descriptions of female rodent sexual behavior can be found in Diakow and Dewsbury (39); McClintock and Adler (25); McClintock, Ansiko, and Adler (40); and Madlafousek and Hlinak (26).

Evaluation of sexual responses in the intact female requires constant and frequent monitoring of individual animals. This is essential because the occurrence of the behavior is restricted to a short and specific period of the ovarian cycle. The behavior normally is expressed only during the time the follicle is undergoing its final preovulatory swelling. The ovarian cycle is usually monitored by taking daily vaginal smears for cytological evaluation, and sexual behavior usually is displayed during the proestrous smear or the transition between proestrous and estrous smears.

The procedure of monitoring the ovarian cycle by daily vaginal smears is cumbersome, time-consuming, and not very precise with respect to the assessment of sexual behavior. When individual females are tested for receptivity and proceptivity at an arbitrary time relative to a particular vaginal cytology, some may be at the beginning of the period of receptivity, some in the middle, and some near the end. Others may not yet have reached the receptive stage, and for those in various segments of the period the quality of receptive behavior will vary accordingly. Furthermore, in the intact female, impairment or absence of sexual response could be due to impairment of pituitary gonadotrophic activity, disordered ovarian production of steroids, or impairment of the response of relevant neural centers to the gonadal hormones.

Undesirable variability as well as uncertainty about the cause of impaired sexual response can be reduced by assessing sexual behavior in spayed females suitably treated with injections of estradiol and progesterone. Usually females are brought into good states of receptivity by a single subcutaneous injection of estradiol benzoate followed 48 hours later with an injection of progesterone. All animals to be tested can then be evaluated at an exact time (usually six hours) after the progesterone injection.

The artificial induction of sexual responses has to be done with precision and with concern for hormonal stimulation that closely approximates the normal physiological pattern. Administration of excessive amounts of estrogen and progesterone could mask or override subtle derangements induced by a toxic substance. If spayed animals are used for assessment of sexual behavior, great care must be exercised to ensure that physiological doses of estrogen and progestagen are administered. Reference to the literature on experimental analysis of female rodent sexual behavior will not be helpful as a guide to proper hormone treatment, since suprathreshold dosage regimens are usually used, and these are not appropriate for screening toxicants. In any attempt to identify damaging actions of a putative toxicant, the investigator should be cautious about exceeding 1 μg of estradiol benzoate and 0.1 mg of progesterone per adult animal. The best general rule to follow is to conduct an initial parametric study on the specific breed or strain to be used and to determine the minimum hormonal requirements for induction of estrous behaviors in a specified percent of the population.

Assessment of human sexual behavior: surveillance and epidemiological studies

Preliminary comments. Direct assessment of human behavior is essential for evaluating the behavioral effects of environmental toxicants. The extrapolation of animal studies to human behavior is limited for a variety of reasons. (a) Many aspects of human sexuality and reproductive behavior are unique and have no obvious animal counterpart (41, 42). (b) While compounds such as steroids do affect sexual motivation in both animals and humans, their behavioral manifestations in humans are often quite different from their manifestations in animals. (c) Human behavior may be disrupted at lower toxicant levels than would be expected from animal studies. (d) The exposure of the general population, but especially workers, to the compound may be greater in fact than originally estimated (also see "Other Considerations").

We present several different methods for assessing the effect of a toxicant on human sexual behavior. Because direct controls may not be possible for practical or ethical reasons, each method has its own weakness. Therefore, we have proposed a variety of methods and suggest that they be used concurrently if at all possible. This extra effort would be justified particularly when the potential benefits of a compound are high, but also when animal toxicological screening or analysis of the compound's structure indicates that the potential risk to human behavior may also be high. In any case, the behavioral assessment procedures for humans need not be cumbersome and can be incorporated in any procedure or physical exam designed to monitor the effects of a putative toxicant on reproductive function.

Behavioral surveillance of humans potentially exposed to a reproductive toxicant. Ideally, new compounds would be released and used at first on a limited basis. Then, changes in sexual satisfaction and function could be assessed prospectively with adequate controls. The sexual experience of the exposed group, perhaps production workers who would be exposed to higher concentrations, could be compared with a matched group of similar workers in an area or plant where the compound was not yet in use. This comparison should be made between two groups of workers in the same plant or location. If this is not possible, the two groups should be matched for factors known to correlate with sexual attitudes and behavior such as socioeconomic status, cohort, ethnicity, religion, and environmental factors. (Industry should use an epidemiologic consultant to determine the matching criteria, sample size, and duration of surveillance appropriate for the amount of natural variance in the proposed measures of sexual behavior.)

If limited release is not warranted ethically or practically and a general release occurs, it would be necessary to monitor sexual satisfaction and the incidence of dysfunction before as well as after the compound is released. The large population variability in normal sexual behavior may make this procedure more sensitive than a comparison between groups. Furthermore, as the behavior of each person is compared to his own normal pattern, it may be possible to identify a subpopulation of particularly sensitive individuals.

These control procedures are essential for evaluating the effect of a toxicant on human sexual behavior, because standard norms are not currently available as a basis for comparison as they are for such physical variables as sperm count or menstrual cycle length. As the number of controlled studies increases, it may be possible to use the data from control groups to develop normative statistics for future evaluations.

The frequency of sexual intercourse is not a good indicator of sexual satisfaction by itself; it is also necessary to evaluate sexual arousal, initiation, and changes in erotic imagery and to identify specific sources of sexual dysfunction. For example, there was little agreement about the nature of changes in women's sexual motivation over the menstrual cycle until studies focused on behavior of the woman herself and her sexual initiation and fantasy rather than on the frequency of intercourse (43, 44).

Either an interview or a short questionnaire can assess sexual satisfaction and function. It is important that the interviewer be trained in interview techniques for sexual counseling. Short courses are currently available for medical and lay personnel in most academic medical centers (Marriage Counseling Center of the University of Pennsylvania has a list). Alternatively, there are a variety of short questionnaires that correlate well with such physiological measures of sexual arousability as penile tumescence and vaginal lubrication (45, 46) and that generate a similar profile whether completion of the questionnaire is mandatory or voluntary (47, 48).

Another approach to the assessment problem is based on epidemiological data. The incidence of cases involving sexual dysfunction reported to such institutions as mental health clinics, local physicians, or plant infirmaries can be recorded and used as a normative data base. This baseline could be compared with the frequency of reported cases following the release of a new compound. Again, an epidemiologic consultant should determine whether the sample from available institutions would be large enough to detect a toxic effect.

Evaluation of human sexual behavior following exposure to a known toxicant. Many compounds have been established as physiological toxicants but have not yet been assessed for behavioral effects in humans. Estrogenic compounds such as DES and DDT may affect the sexuality of women, while organopesticides that are neurotoxins, such as carbaryl, an acetylcholine esterase inhibitor, may affect male erectile function.

If a population has been exposed to such compounds or is suspected of being at reproductive risk, behavioral assessment can be made at the time that a physiological assessment is being made. The same personnel could do this, provided that they have been trained in interview techniques. Behavioral assessment under these *ex post facto* conditions is particularly difficult because knowledge of exposure to a toxicant can distort the retrospective assessment of sexual satisfaction and behavior. Therefore, trained personnel, an evaluation immediately after the exposure, and established norms would each help to reduce this bias. In any event, an unexposed control population should be evaluated using the identical retrospective procedures and matched to the target population for such variables as socioeconomic status, ethnic group, and local environment.

Risk assessment. If any significant alterations are found, exposure to the toxicant should be discontinued to assess the reversibility of the effects. Furthermore, the mechanism of action will need to be identified to evaluate a risk/benefit ratio. For example, it is possible that erectile function could be impaired through a direct impairment of cholinergic mechanisms or indirectly through an increase in depression or sense of fatigue (49). Nocturnal penile tumescence would aid in a differential diagnosis, as erectile function during sleep is not impaired by psychogenic factors. Human sexuality is particularly sensitive to disruption by many environmental and psychological factors that are not specifically sexual themselves; most instances of sexual dysfunction encountered in the clinic are not the result of a direct organic cause. Therefore, the mechanisms of any impairment of sexual performance or satisfaction will have to be determined before a risk/benefit ratio can be assessed.

Priority areas for future research

Few experimental studies have been made of the effects of toxic substances on the sexual behavior of laboratory animals. A few recent references (50–61) are included in the listing at the end of this chapter, but they deal primarily with effects of drugs like cannabis, alcohol, and morphine. A search of the literature between

1978 and 1980 revealed only two references dealing with other agents, one on cyanogenic substances (62) and the other on lindane (63). In addition, no systematic evaluations of sexual behavior have been conducted on humans known to have been exposed to toxic substances either in adulthood or prenatally. This unfortunate circumstance, that parallel studies have not been carried out on intentionally exposed animal subjects and on accidentally exposed human beings, severely limits the capability to formulate either qualitative or quantitative risk assessments for sexual functioning.

Basic research on human sexual behavior should be strongly encouraged at this time so that appropriate demographic norms and standards can be established. Adequate information on these matters has not been developed despite the pioneering efforts of Kinsey in the late forties. In addition, changes in concepts, data gathering techniques, and attitudes require modernization of the data base. As pointed out in earlier sections of this discussion, neither measurement of number of offspring produced, frequency of coitus, or even frequency of orgasm are adequate as indicators of human sexual functioning. There is a strong need to develop epidemiological studies of human sexual behavior in its broadest scope and in terms most meaningful to human welfare and to the stability of interpersonal relationships.

The scope of investigations of animal sexual behavior should be broadened. Efforts to establish models permitting better measurement of sexual attractiveness, sexual motivation or desire, and even sexual gratification should be encouraged. Moreover, sound parametric data on the effects of known environmental toxicants ought to be vigorously pursued. These studies could be carried out profitably at this time even with the limited number of behavioral measures currently available, and there should be strong support for such studies on a variety of species. The limitation of data bases, no matter how extensive, to rats and guinea pigs poses a serious obstacle to flexible choice of alternative models that may in fact be more appropriate to human problems.

Finally, even from the relatively limited standpoint of sexual behavior, more information is needed on how different classes of chemical substances interact with central neural tissues on the cellular levels. Information of this sort is fundamental not only to interpretation of toxicant effects on behavior, but also to sound hypothesis formulation and to development of a framework that would permit prediction of the likely biological effects of a putative toxicant.

REFERENCES

1. Rausch, L., Klein, J., Shaffer, S. Q. and Stein, Z.: Effect of chlorination of drinking water on perinatal mortality in New York villages, 1968-1977. Abstract. Am. J. Epidemiol. 112: 439, 1980.

2. Levine, R. J., Symons, M. J., Balogh, S. A., Arndt, D. M., Kaswandik, N. T. and Gentile, J. W.: A method for monitoring the fertility of workers: I. Method and pilot studies. J. Occup. Med. 22: 781–791, 1980.

3. Levine, R. J., Symons, M. J., Balogh, S. A., Milby, T. H. and Whorton, M. D.: A method for monitoring the fertility of workers. II. Validation of the method among workers exposed to dibromochloropropane. J. Occup. Med. 23: 183–188, 1981.

4. Slone, D., Shapiro, S. and Miettinen, O. S.: Case-control surveillance of serious illnesses attributable to ambulatory drug use. In: Epidemiological Evaluation of Drugs, F. Colombo, S. Shapiro, D. Slone, and G. Tognoni, Eds., Elsevier North-Holland Biomedical Press: Amsterdam; pp. 59–82, 1977.

5. Rosenberg, L., Shapiro, S., Slone, D., Kaufman, D. W., Miettinen, O. S. and Stolley, P. D.: Thiazides and acute cholecystits. N. Engl. J. Med. 303: 546–548, 1980.

6. Mitchell, A. A., Rosenberg, L., Shapiro, S. and Slone, D.: Birth defects related to use of Bendictine in pregnancy. I. Oral clefts and cardiac defects. J. Am. Med. Assoc. 245: 2311–2314, 1981.

7. Selikoff, I. J., Churg, J. and Hammond, E. C.: Relation between exposure to asbestos and mesothelioma. New Engl. J. Med. 272: 560–565, 1965.

8. Lee, A. M. and Fraumeni, J. F., Jr.: Arsenic and respiratory cancer in man: An occupational study. J. Natl. Cancer Inst. 42: 1045–1052, 1969.

9. Harlap, S., Shiono, P., Ramcharan, S., Berendes, H. and Pellegrin, F.: A prospective study of spontaneous fetal losses after induced abortions. New Engl. J. Med. 301: 677–681, 1979.

10. Notari, R. E.: Biopharmaceutics and Pharmacokinetics: An Introduction. 3rd Edition, Marcel Dekker: New York; 329 pp., 1980.

11. Wagner, J. G.: Biopharmaceutics and relevant pharmacokinetics. Drug Intelligence Publications: Washington, D.C.; 375 pp., 1971.

12. Gibaldi, M. and Perrier, D.: Pharmacokinetics. Marcel Dekker: New York; 325 pp., 1975.

13. Bischoff, K. B.: Some fundamental considerations of the application of pharmacokinetics to cancer chemotherapy. Cancer Chemother. Rep. Part 1 59: 777–796, 1975.

14. Himmelstein, K. J. and Lutz, R. J.: A review of the applications of physiologically based pharmacokinetic modeling. J. Pharmacokinet. Biopharm. 7: 127–145, 1979.

15. Dedrick, R. L.: Animal scale-up. J. Pharmacokinet. Biopharm. 1: 435–461, 1973.

16. Dedrick, R. L. and Bischoff, K. B.: Species similarities in pharmacokinetics. Fed. Proc. 39: 54–59, 1980.

17. Gehring, P. J., Watanabe, P. G. and Blau, G. E.: Pharmacokinetic studies in evaluation of the toxicological and environmental hazard of chemicals: In: Advances in Modern Toxicology: New Concepts in Safety Evaluation, M. Mehlman, H. Blumenthal, and R. Shapiro, Eds., Hemisphere Publishing Corporation: New York; pp. 195–290, 1976.

18. World Health Organization. Chemobiokinetics and metabolism. In: Environmental Health Criteria 6. Principles and Methods for Evaluating the Toxicity of Chemicals. Geneva; pp. 116–177, 1978.

19. Filov, V. A., Golubev, A. A., Liublina, E. I. and Tolokontsev, N. A.: Quantitative Toxicology. John Wiley: New York; 462 pp., 1980.

20. Young, J. F. and Holson, J. F.: Utility of pharmacokinetics in designing toxicological protocols and improving interspecies extrapolation. J. Environ. Pathol. Toxicol. 2: 169–186, 1978.

21. Souchay, A. M., Rice, P. C., Rourke, J. E. and Nesbitt, R. E. L.: Glucose metabolism and transfer in the human placenta. In: Chemical Engineering in Medicine, D. D. Reneau, Ed., Plenum Press: New York; pp. 172–199, 1973.

22. Dedrick, R. L., Meyers, C. E., Bungay, P. M. and De Vita, V. T.: Pharmacokinetic rationale for peritoneal drug administration in the treatment of ovarian cancer. Cancer Treatment Rep. 62: 1–11, 1978.

23. Lee, I. P. and Dixon, R. L.: Factors influencing reproduction and genetic toxic effects on male gonads. Environ. Health Perspect. 24: 117–127, 1978.

24. Beach, F. A.: Animal models for human sexuality. In: CIBA Foundation Symposium, No. 62. Sex, Hormones, and Behavior, Mar. 14–16, 1978, London, England, Elsevier-North Holland: New York; pp. 133–144, 1979.

25. McClintock, M. K. and Adler, N. T.: The role of the female during copulation in wild and domestic rats (*Rattus norvegicus*). Behavior 67: 67–96, 1978.

26. Madlafousek, J. and Hlinak, Z.: Sexual behavior of the female laboratory rat: inventory, patterning, and measurement. Behavior 63: 129–174, 1977.

27. Dewsbury, D. A.: A quantitative description of the behavior of rats during copulation. Behaviour 29: 154–178, 1967.

28. Dewsbury, D. A.: Description of sexual behavior in research on hormone-behavior interactions. In: Endocrine Control of Sexual Behavior, C. Beyer, Ed., New York: Raven Press, pp. 3–32, 1979.

29. McClintock, M. K., Toner, J. P., Adler, N. T. and Anisko, J. J.: Postejaculatory quiescence in female and male rats: consequences for sperm transport during group mating. J. Comp. Physiol. Psychol.; in press, 1982.

30. Beach, F. A. and Jordan, L.: Sexual exhaustion and recovery in the male rat. Q. J. Exp. Psychol. 8: 121–133, 1956.

31. Larsson, K.: Conditioning and Sexual Behavior in the Male Albino Rat. Stockholm: Almquist & Wiksell; 1956.

32. Sachs, B. D. and Barfield, R.: Functional analysis of masculine copulatory behavior in the rat. Adv. Study Behav. 7: 91–154, 1976.

33. Young, W. C.: Psychobiology of sexual behavior in the guinea pig. Adv. Study Behav. 2: 1–110, 1969.

34. Young, W. C. and Grunt, J. A.: The pattern and measurement of sexual behavior in the male guinea pig. J. Comp. Physiol. Psychol. 44: 492–500, 1951.

35. Dewsbury, D. A.: Copulatory behavior of rats: Variations within the dark phase of the diurnal cycle. Commun. Behav. Biol. 1: 373–377, 1968.

36. Fadem, B. H., Barfield, R. J. and Whalen, R. E.: Dose-response and time-response relationships between progesterone and the display of patterns of receptive and proceptive behavior in the female rat. Horm. Behav. 13: 40–48, 1979.

37. Goy, R. W. and Young, W. C.: Strain differences in the behavioral responses of female guinea pigs to alpha-estradiol benzoate and progesterone. Behaviour 10: 340–354, 1957.

38. Walker, W. A. and Feder, H. H.: The comparative potency of various steroids to complete the priming process for lordosis in guinea pigs. Horm. Behav. 12: 299–308, 1979.

39. Diakow, C. and Dewsbury, D. A.: A compuative description of the mating behavior of female rodents. Anim. Behav. 26: 1091–1097, 1978.

40. McClintock, M. K., Anisko, J. J. and Adler, N. T.: Group mating among Norway rats. I. Sex differences in the pattern and neuroendocrine consequences of copulation. Anim. Behav.; in press, 1982.

41. Beach, F. A.: Cross-species comparisons and the human heritage. In: Human Sexuality in Four Perspectives, F. A. Beach, Ed., Johns Hopkins University Press: Baltimore; pp., 296–316, 1977.

42. Beach, F. A.: Animal models and psychological inference. In: Human Sexuality: A Developmental and Comparative Approach, H. A. Katchadourian, Ed., University of California Press: Berkeley; pp. 98–112, 1979.

43. Adams, D., Gold, A. and Burt A.: Rise in female-initiated sexual activity at ovulation and its suppression by oral contraceptives. N. Engl. J. Med. 299: 1145–1150, 1978.

44. Persky, H., Lief, H., Strauss, D., Miller, W. and O'Brien, C. D.: Plasma testosterone level and sexual behavior of couples. Arch. Sex. Behav. 7: 157–173, 1978.

45. Byrne, D. and Scheffield, J.: Response to sexually arousing stimuli as a function of repressing and sensitizing defenses. J. Abnorm. Psychol. 70: 114–118, 1965.

46. Byrne, D., Fisher, J. D., Lamberth, J. and Mitchell, H. E.: Evaluations of erotica: Facts or feelings. J. Pers. Soc. Psychol. 29: 111–116, 1974.

47. Kaats, A. and Davis, K.: Effects of volunteer biases in studies of sexual behavior and attitudes. J. Sex. Res. 7: 219–227, 1971.

48. Bauman, K.: Volunteer bias in a study of sexual knowledge, attitudes, and behavior. J. Marr. Fam. 35: 27–31, 1975.

49. Kaplan, H. S.: The New Sex Therapy, Brunner/Mazel: New York; 544 pp., 1974.

50. Abel, E. L.: A review of alcohol's effects on sex and reproduction. Drug Alcohol Depend. 5: 321–332, 1980.

51. Barnes, T. R., Bamber, R. W. and Watson, J. P.: Psychotropic drugs and sexual behaviour. Br. J. Hosp. Med. 21: 594–600, 1979.

52. Clemens, L. G., Popham, T. V. and Ruppert, P. H.: Neonatal treatment of hamsters with barbiturate alters adult sexual behavior. Dev. Psychobiol. 12: 49–59, 1979.

53. Dalterio, S. L.: Perinatal or adult exposure to cannabinoids alters male reproductive functions in mice. Pharmacol. Biochem. Behav. 12: 143–153, 1980.

54. Dalterio, S. and Bartke, A.: Perinatal exposure to cannabinoids alters male reproductive function in mice. Science 205: 1420–1422, 1979.

55. Gordon, J. H., Bromley, B. L., Gorski, R. A. and Zimmermann, E.: Delta9-tetrahydrocannabinol enhancement of lordosis behavior in estrogen treated female rats. Pharmacol. Biochem. Behav. 8: 603–608, 1978.

56. Kostellow, A. B., Ziegler, D., Kunar, J., Fujimoto, G. I. and Morrill, G. A.: Effect of cannabinoids on estrous cycle, ovulation, and reproductive capacity of female A/J mice. Pharmacology 21: 68–75, 1980.

57. Kumar, R., Mumford, L. and Teixeira, A. R.: Sexual behavior in morphine-dependent rats [proceedings]. Br. J. Pharmacol. 62: 389P–390P, 1978.

58. Mumford, L. and Kumar, R.: Sexual behaviour of morphine-dependent and abstinent male rats. Psychopharmacologie (Berlin) 65: 179–185, 1979.

59. Ostrowski, N. L., Stapleton, J. M., Noble, R. G. and Reid, L. D.: Morphine and naloxone's effects on sexual behavior of the female golden hamster. Pharmacol. Biochem. Behav. 11: 673–681, 1979.

60. Rosenkrantz, H.: Effects on cannabis on fetal development of rodents. Adv. Biosci. 22–23: 479–499, 1978.

61. Vorhees, C. V., Brunner, R. L. and Butcher, R. E.: Psychotropic drugs as behavioral teratogens. Science 205: 1220–1225, 1979.

62. Olusi, S. O., Oke, O. L. and Odusote, A.: Effects of cyanogenic agents on reproduction and neonatal development in rats. Biol. Neonate 36: 233–243, 1979.

63. Palmer, A. K., Cozens, D. D., Spicer, E. J. and Worden, A. N.: Effects of lindane upon reproductive function in a three-generation study in rats. Toxicology 10: 45–54, 1978.

STEERING COMMITTEE

K. Diane Courtney, Ph.D.
Research Pharmacologist
Pesticides and Toxic Substances
  Effects Laboratory
U.S. Environmental Protection
  Agency
Research Triangle Park, NC 27711

Wayne M. Galbraith, Ph.D.†
Toxicologist
Office of Research and Development
U.S. Environmental Protection
  Agency
Washington, D.C. 20460
(EPA Co–Project Officer)

Richard M. Hoar, Ph.D.
Head of Teratology and Assistant
  Director of Toxicology
Department of Toxicology
Hoffmann–LaRoche, Inc.
Nutley, NJ 07110
(Chairman of Reproduction
  Groups)

E. Marshall Johnson, Ph.D.
Professor and Chairman
Department of Anatomy
Director, Daniel Baugh Institute
  of Anatomy
Jefferson Medical College
Thomas Jefferson University
Philadelphia, PA 19107
(Chairman of Developmental Group)

Robert M. Pratt, Ph.D.*
Chief, Experimental Teratogenesis
  Section
Laboratory of Reproductive &
  Developmental Toxicology
National Institute of Environmental
  Health Sciences
National Institutes of Health
Research Triangle Park, NC 27709

Michael G. Ryon, M.S.
Information Analyst
Chemical Effects Information
  Center
Oak Ridge National Laboratory
Oak Ridge, TN 37830

Peter Voytek, Ph.D.
Director, Reproductive Effects
  Assessment Group
Office of Research and
  Development
U.S. Environmental Protection
  Agency
Washington, D.C. 20460
(EPA Co–Project Officer)

Rupert P. Amann, Ph.D.
Professor of Physiology and
  Biophysics
Animal Reproduction Laboratory
Colorado State University
Fort Collins, CO 80525

J. Michael Bedford, Ph.D.
Professor of Obstetrics and
  Gynecology and of Anatomy
Cornell Medical School
New York, NY 10021
(Chairman of Male Reproduction
  Group)

Allan R. Beaudoin, Ph.D.
Assistant Chairman and Professor
Department of Anatomy
University of Michigan Medical
  School
Ann Arbor, MI 48104

Kenneth B. Bischoff, Ph.D.
Chairman, Department of Chemical
  Engineering
Professor of Biomedical and
  Chemical Engineering
University of Delaware
Newark, DE 19711

William J. Bremner, M.D., Ph.D.
Chief, Endocrinology Section
Veterans Administration Medical
  Center
Associate Professor of Medicine
  and of Obstetrics and Gynecology
University of Washington School
  of Medicine
Seattle, WA 98108

Charles C. Brown, Ph.D.*
Statistician, Biometry Branch
National Cancer Institute
Bethesda, MD 20205

Mildred S. Christian, Ph.D.
Director of Research
Argus Research Laboratories
Perkasie, PA 18944

James H. Clark, Ph.D.
Professor of Cell Biology
Baylor College of Medicine
Houston, TX 77030
(Chairman of Female
  Reproduction Group)

Thomas F. X. Collins, Ph.D.
Chief, Mammalian Reproduction
  and Teratology
Division of Toxicology
Bureau of Foods
Food and Drug Administration
Washington, D.C. 20204

Donald A. Dewsbury, Ph.D.*
Professor of Psychology
University of Florida
Gainesville, FL 32611

Larry L. Ewing, Ph.D.*
Professor of Reproduction
  Biology
School of Hygiene and Public
  Health
Johns Hopkins University
Baltimore, MD 21205

---

*Attended only the St. Louis workshop.

148

Robert H. Foote, Ph.D.
Professor of Animal Science
Cornell University
Ithaca, NY 14850

David W. Gaylor, Ph.D.
Director, Division of Biometry
National Center for Toxicological
  Research
Jefferson, AR 72079

Arnold A. Gerall, Ph.D.*
Professor of Psychology
Tulane University
New Orleans, LA 70118

Robert W. Goy, Ph.D.*
Director, Wisconsin Regional
  Primate Research Center
University of Wisconsin
Madison, WI 53706
(Chairman of Behavior Group)

Arthur F. Haney, M.D.
Assistant Professor of Obstetrics
  and Gynecology
Duke University Medical Center
Durham, NC 27710

W. LeRoy Heinrichs, Ph.D., M.D.*
Chairman and Professor
Department of Gynecology and
  Obstetrics
Stanford University
Stanford, CA 94305

Mary C. Henry, Ph.D.*
Research Pharmacologist
Environmental Protection Research
  Division
U.S. Army Biomedical Engineering
  Research and Development
  Laboratory
Fort Detrick
Frederick, MD 21701

Jerry Highfill, M.S.
Statistician, Health Effects
  Research Laboratory
U.S. Environmental Protection
  Agency
Research Triangle Park, NC 27711

Carol J. Hogue, Ph.D.
Associate Professor of Biometry
University of Arkansas for
  Medical Sciences
Little Rock, AR 72201

Donald E. Hutchings, Ph.D.
Research Scientist
Department of Behavioral
  Physiology
New York State Psychiatric
  Institute
Assistant Professor of Medical
  Psychology
Department of Pediatrics
Columbia University
New York, NY 10031

Harold Kalter, Ph.D.
Research Associate
Children's Hospital Research
  Foundation
Professor of Research
Department of Pediatrics
University of Cincinnati
Cincinnati, OH 45229

---

*Attended only the St. Louis workshop.

Carole A. Kimmel, Ph.D.*
Chief, Perinatal and Postnatal
  Evaluation Branch
Research Pharmacologist
Division of Teratogenesis
  Research
National Center for Toxicological
  Research
Jefferson, AR 72079

Devendra M. Kochhar, Ph.D.
Professor of Anatomy
Jefferson Medical College
Thomas Jefferson University
Philadelphia, PA 19107

Donna Kuroda, Ph.D.
Physical Sciences Administrator
Reproductive Effects
  Assessment Group
U.S. Environmental Protection
  Agency
Washington, D.C. 20460

Donald R. Mattison, M.D.
Medical Officer
Pregnancy Research Branch
National Institute of Child
  Health and Human Development
National Institutes of Health
Bethesda, MD 20205

Martha K. McClintock, Ph.D.*
Assistant Professor of Behavioral
  Sciences
University of Chicago
Chicago, IL 60637

Wilbur P. McNulty, M.D.
Chairman, Laboratory of Pathology
Oregon Regional Primate Research
  Center
Beaverton, OR 97006

Marvin L. Meistrich, Ph.D.
Associate Professor of
  Experimental Radiotherapy
University of Texas System
  Cancer Center
M.D. Anderson Hospital Tumor
  Institute
Houston, TX 77030

Eugene F. Oakberg, Ph.D.*
Senior Research Staff Member
Mammalian Genetics and
  Development Section
Biology Division
Oak Ridge National Laboratory
Oak Ridge, TN 37830

James W. Overstreet, Ph.D., M.D.*
Associate Professor of Human
  Anatomy and of Obstetrics and
  Gynecology
University of California, Davis
  Medical School
Davis, CA 95616

John C. Porter, Ph.D.
Professor of Physiology and of
  Obstetrics and Gynecology
University of Texas Health Science
  Center at Dallas
Southwestern Medical School
Dallas, TX 75235

Lynn Rosenberg, Sc.D.
Assistant Research Professor
Boston University
Biostatistician and
  Epidemiologist
Drug Epidemiology Unit
Boston University Medical
  Center
Cambridge, MA 02138

---

*Attended only the St. Louis workshop.

Griff T. Ross, Ph.D., M.D.†
Deputy Director of the
 Clinical Center
National Institutes of Health
Bethesda, MD 20205

Liane B. Russell, Ph.D.†
Head of Mammalian Genetics and
 Teratology Section
Biology Division
Oak Ridge National Laboratory
Oak Ridge, TN 37830

Carol Sakai, Ph.D.
Reproductive Toxicologist
Reproductive Effects Assessment
 Group
Office of Research and
 Development
U.S. Environmental Protection
 Agency
Washington, D.C. 20460

Thomas H. Shepard, M.D.*
Professor of Pediatrics
Head, Central Laboratory for
 Human Embryology
University of Washington
Seattle, WA 98195

Richard G. Skalko, Ph.D.
Professor and Chairman
Department of Anatomy
College of Medicine
East Tennessee State University
Johnson City, TN 37614

Kate Smith, Ph.D.*
Developmental Toxicologist
Health Effects Research Laboratory
U.S. Environmental Protection
 Agency
Cincinnati, OH 45268

Robert E. Staples, Ph.D.
Staff Teratologist
Haskell Laboratory (DuPont)
Wilmington, DE 19898

Robert G. Tardiff, Ph.D.†
Executive Director, Board on
 Toxicology and Environmental
 Health Hazards
National Academy of Sciences
Washington, D.C. 20418

William J. Waddell, M.D.
Professor and Chairman
Department of Pharmacology and
 Toxicology
School of Medicine
University of Louisville
Louisville, KY 40292

Ronald J. Young, Ph.D.
Associate Professor and Research
 Associate
Department of Obstetrics and
 Gynecology
Cornell University Medical College
New York, NY 10021

---

*Attended only the St. Louis workshop.
†Attended only the Atlanta workshop.

REVIEWERS

The assistance of the following persons in the review process is gratefully acknowledged. The final content of the report is the responsibility of the steering committee and the group chairmen.

Aaron Blair, Ph.D.
Environmental Epidemiology
  Branch
National Institutes of Health

Joseph Borzelleca, Ph.D.
Department of Pharmacology
Medical College of Virginia

Robert Dedrick, Ph.D.
Biomedical Engineering and
  Instrumentation Branch
National Institutes of Health

James Emerson, Ph.D.
Life Sciences
Coca Cola Company

Michael Farrow, Ph.D.
Genetic Toxicology Department
Hazleton Laboratories America,
  Inc.

Ernst Freese, Ph.D.
Laboratory of Molecular Biology
National Institutes of Health

Vera Glocklin, Ph.D.
Bureau of Drugs
U.S. Food and Drug Administration

Andrew G. Hendrickx, Ph.D.
California Primate Research
  Center
University of California, Davis

Kundan S. Khera, Ph.D.
Health Protection Branch
Health and Welfare Canada

Renate Kimbrough, M.D.
Toxicology Branch
Centers for Disease Control

George Levinskas, Ph.D.
Environmental Assessment and
  Toxicology
Monsanto Company

Lawrence B. Mellett, Ph.D.
Scientific Liaison and Compliance
Revlon Health Care Group

Roy Mundy, Ph.D.
Department of Pharmacology
University of Alabama,
  Birmingham

Frederick Oehme, D.V.M., Ph.D.
Comparative Toxicology Laboratory
Kansas State University

Anthony K. Palmer
Huntingdon Research Centre

Bobby Joe Payne, D.V.M., Ph.D.
Director of Pathology
Toxicity Research Laboratories,
  Ltd.

Harold M. Peck, M.D.
Safety Assessment
Merck Institute for Therapeutic
  Research

David Rall, M.D., Ph.D.
National Institute of Environmental
  and Health Sciences

Robert Scala, Ph.D.
Medical and Environmental Health
　Department
Exxon Corporation

Charlotte Schneyer, Ph.D.
Laboratory of Exocrine Physiology
University of Alabama,
　Birmingham

Bernard A. Schwetz, D.V.M., Ph.D.
Health and Environmental
　Sciences
Dow Chemical U.S.A.

Marshall Steinberg, Ph.D.
Life Sciences Division
Hazleton Laboratories America, Inc.

Clarence J. Terhaar, Ph.D.
Toxicology Section
Eastman Kodak Company

Hanspeter Witschi, M.D.
Biology Division
Oak Ridge National Laboratory

Gerhard Zbindin, M.D.
Institute of Toxicology

INDEX

abstinence interval, 60, 82
acceptable daily intake (ADI), 9,
    48, 56, 110
acceptable dosage level, 48, 111,
    112
accessory sex glands, 6, 47 (Table 8),
    49 (Table 9), 50 (Table 10), 51,
    60, 73, 75-77, 79, 84
acute, 3, 57, 70, 71, 99, 122
adenosis, 8 (Table 1), 37
adolescence, 126
adrenal, 8 (Table 1), 127
adult toxic dose, 108, 111, 112
age, 7, 10, 11, 14 (Table 2), 16,
    19-21, 28, 48 (Table 8), 50
    (Table 10), 52, 53, 60, 74, 75,
    82, 111, 118
amenorrhea, 20, 37, 39
androgen, 5, 6, 14, 19, 20, 30, 33
    (Table 6), 37, 62, 73, 93, 126,
    128-130
animal
  model, 11, 17, 18, 20, 23, 28,
    30,32, 41-43, 44 (Table 7),
    50 (Table 10), 52, 56, 57, 58
    (Table 11), 60, 62, 69, 71, 83,
    110 (Table 12), 122, 124,
    128-130, 140
  testing, 2, 6, 13, 19, 22, 25-27,
    42, 46, 47 (Table 8), 49
    (Table 9), 50 (Table 10), 52,
    55-57, 58 (Table 11), 59-61,
    81, 85, 86, 100, 101, 104, 106,
    108, 109, 110 (Table 12), 111,
    112, 119, 130-137, 139, 140
anovulation, 8 (Table 1), 17, 20, 37
artificial insemination, 43, 44
    (Table 7), 58 (Table 11), 85

attractivity, 124, 125, 131, 134,
    135, 140
azoospermia, 54, 59

bioaccumulation, 48, 57, 58
    (Table 11), 59, 102, 108
breast, 8 (Table 1)

case-control study, 118-120
cauda epididymidis, 44 (Table 7),
    49, 51, 59, 72, 74, 83
cell culture, 22-24, 31, 32, 33
    (Table 6), 62, 109, 110
    (Table 12)
chronic, 8 (Table 1), 46, 48
    (Table 8), 51, 70, 71, 88, 99,
    111, 122
cleft lip, 101
cleft palate, 101
coefficient of variation (CV), 46,
    50 (Table 10), 60, 62, 75, 77, 81
cohort-studies, 118, 119, 121, 137
computerized integrated data base,
    4 (Fig. 1), 5-7, 9, 10, 121
conception, 43, 118
conceptive ability, 6, 17, 31
conceptus, 1, 99, 100, 103, 104,
    106-110, 112, 122
congenital defects (or malforma-
    tions), 100, 118
control groups, 16, 46, 53-57, 61,
    70-72, 74, 77, 78, 80-84, 123,
    132, 137-139
copulation plug, 16
copulatory behavior, 17, 132-134

corpus luteum (lutea), 17, 30, 32,
37, 47 (Table 8), 50 (Table 10),
83, 85
correlational studies, 118
cost/benefit, 16, 17, 49 (Table 9),
108, 139
critical periods of development,
20, 102, 103

decidual implantation, 104, 105
demographic studies, 3, 118
developmental abnormalities (or
defects or malformations), 99,
100, 103-107, 110 (Table 12),
118, 126, 129, 130
developmental toxic dose, 108,
110 (Table 12), 111, 112
diestrus, 20, 37
DNA, 31, 49 (Table 9), 62, 87
dog, 43, 44 (Table 7), 79, 131
domestic animals, 32, 42, 43, 46,
70, 74, 76, 79, 107, 108
dopamine, 11, 21, 24, 37
dose, 6, 16, 18-20, 22, 26, 27,
47 (Table 8), 51, 52, 55-57,
59, 61, 83, 87, 88, 95, 101-104,
106-109, 111, 121, 122, 130,
134, 136
dose-response (relationship), 2, 9,
18, 20, 23, 24, 26-28, 47 (Table 8),
48, 57, 79, 85, 87, 88, 101, 103,
109-111, 112 (Table 12), 119
ductus deferens, 72

ejaculate, 41-43, 46, 47 (Table 10),
49, 50 (Table 10), 51, 54, 55, 59,
60, 69, 73-79, 82, 84, 85, 87, 94,
133
ejaculation, 42, 43, 44 (Table 7),
51, 60, 74, 76, 77, 94, 132, 133
embryo, 47 (Table 8), 50 (Table 10),
59, 83, 85, 86, 101-103, 105,
109, 110 (Table 12), 112

embryonic development, 41, 62,
102-105
emission, 95
endocrine, 1, 26, 43, 46, 47
(Table 8), 50 (Table 10), 53, 79,
80, 103, 105, 107, 126, 134
epidemiology (epidemiologic), 1,
3, 5, 12, 53, 56, 106, 117, 119-
121, 136-138, 140
epididymis, 41, 46, 47 (Table 8),
49 (Table 9), 50 (Table 10), 51,
59, 70, 72-75, 78, 83, 84
estradiol, 14, 18, 19, 22, 26, 33
(Table 6), 37, 127, 129, 134,
136
estrogen, 5, 9, 11, 13, 14 (Table 2),
18, 19, 21, 23, 25-27, 30, 33
(Table 6), 37, 38, 126-129, 136,
138
estrogenicity, 5, 6, 9, 11, 13, 14,
18, 19, 21-23, 27
estrus, 14, 15 (Table 3), 16, 17,
20, 38, 104, 133, 134, 136
extrapolation, 10-12, 18-20, 30,
32, 56, 100, 102, 104, 111, 112,
117, 122, 123, 130, 136

fallopian tubes, 8 (Table 1)
false negative, 16, 17, 109
false positive, 5, 17, 109
fecundity, 17
fertility, 16, 17, 28, 41-43, 44
(Table 7), 46, 47 (Table 8), 50
(Table 10), 51, 53-56, 59, 60,
78, 83-87, 107, 118, 120
fertilization, 41, 43, 62
fetal development, 10, 14, 20, 62,
102-105, 129
fetus, 2, 5, 102, 105, 106, 122,
129, 130
follicle, 11, 21, 28, 29 (Table 4),
30, 32, 33 (Table 6), 38, 135
follicle-stimulating hormone (FSH),
21, 30, 38, 41, 47 (Table 8), 50
(Table 10), 53, 54, 59, 61, 62,
79-84, 95

gamete, 8 (Table 1), 27, 28, 104
germ cell, 49 (Table 9), 71, 74
germinal epithelium, 49, 54, 57,
    59, 69, 71, 73, 78
gestation, 8 (Table 1), 18, 20,
    102-104
gonad, 30, 54, 104, 122, 124, 126,
    128, 136
gonadotropin, 10, 17, 21, 22, 26,
    30-32, 38, 136
gonadotropin-releasing hormone
    (GnRH), 21, 22, 24, 47 (Table 8),
    50 (Table 10), 54, 61, 80, 82
granulosa, 30, 32, 33 (Table 6)
gross anatomical (or structural)
    defects, 106, 107
guinea pig, 17, 27, 127-129, 131,
    133-135, 140

hamster, 43, 47 (Table 8), 82, 84,
    86, 87, 127, 129
hazard, 1, 6, 41-43, 53, 62, 69, 85,
    99, 100, 106, 108, 109, 111,
    112, 117-121
heterospermic insemination, 62
hormone, 5, 6, 8 (Table 1), 9, 11,
    21, 25, 27, 30, 33 (Table 6),
    41, 44 (Table 7), 47 (Table 8),
    50 (Table 10), 53, 54, 59, 61,
    62, 79-84, 95, 124, 126-131,
    133, 136
human, 1-3, 5-7, 9-12, 16-20, 22,
    24, 27, 28, 30-32, 41-43, 44
    (Table 7), 47 (Table 8), 49
    (Table 9), 50 (Table 10), 52-62,
    70, 75, 76, 79-82, 84-88, 99-
    102, 106-112, 117, 119, 120,
    122-130, 134-140
human chorionic gonadotropin
    (HCG), 31
hypothalamus (hypothalamic), 5,
    8 (Table 1), 11, 20, 21, 24-27,
    38, 80, 128, 131
hypothesis-generating studies,
    117-119

implantation, 14, 104
infertility, 1, 5, 42, 43, 52, 54, 55,
    80, 82, 118
intromission, 132, 133
in utero, 104, 106
in vitro, 10, 18, 22-24, 30, 32, 33
    (Table 6), 44 (Table 7), 47
    (Table 8), 61, 62, 79, 82, 84,
    85, 109, 110 (Table 12)
in vivo, 10, 14, 18, 19, 21-23, 30,
    31, 57, 62, 79, 85, 86, 108, 109

lactation, 6, 8 (Table 1), 14, 16,
    18, 38, 104, 105
leydig cell, 61, 62, 72
libido, 20, 43, 84, 124, 127, 132,
    140
litter size, 18, 84
live birth index, 18
lordosis, 26, 27, 135
luteinizing hormone (LH), 21, 22,
    25, 30, 38, 41, 47 (Table 8),
    50 (Table 10), 54, 59, 61, 62,
    79-84, 95

masculinization, 5, 10, 20, 40,
    126, 129
maternal-fetal exchange, 102
maternal toxicity, 110
mating, 14, 15 (Table 3), 16, 17,
    26, 27, 44 (Table 7), 46, 58
    (Table 11), 59, 62, 83, 85, 86,
    104, 133
mating behavior, 14, 20, 25, 26
maximum tolerated dose (MTD),
    16, 47 (Table 8), 49 (Table 9),
    57, 83, 88, 95
menopause, 8 (Table 1), 28, 38
menstruation, 17, 30, 138
model system, 9-11, 28, 32, 43,
    60, 69, 71, 101, 110 (Table 12),
    122, 124, 130
motility (or motile), 42, 43, 46,
    47 (Table 8), 50 (Table 10), 51,
    53, 60, 72, 73, 75, 77-79, 82-84, 95

mounts, 124, 126, 132, 133, 135
mouse (mice), 6, 11, 28, 43, 44
    (Table 7), 51, 61, 74, 102, 110
    (Table 12), 127, 129
multigenerational, 6, 15 (Table 3),
    104, 105

nonmotile spermatozoan, 95
no-observed-effect level (NOEL)
    or (no-adverse-effect level), 56,
    103, 110

oligomenorrhea, 20, 38
oligozoospermia, 54
oocyte, 8 (Table 1), 11, 18, 27,
    28, 29 (Table 4), 39, 84
oogenesis, 28
oral contraceptive, 11
organogenesis, 101, 102, 105,
    106, 122
ovary, 8 (Table 1), 16-18, 21, 25,
    27, 28, 30-32, 33 (Table 6),
    127, 134-136
ovotoxicity, 11
ovulation, 10, 14, 17, 20, 21, 39

parturition, 8 (Table 1), 39
pharmacokinetics, 1, 56, 101,
    103, 111, 112, 117, 121-123,
    130
phenotypic transformation, 20
pituitary, 8 (Table 1), 10, 21-26,
    54, 80, 128
placenta, 8 (Table 1), 102, 103,
    112, 129, 130
placental transfer, 8 (Table 1), 102
population-based registries, 118
postpartum, 14, 15 (Table 3), 16
potency, 18, 19, 22, 23, 128
pregnancy, 5, 6, 8 (Table 1), 16,
    20, 47 (Table 8), 50 (Table 10),
    52, 105, 110, 117, 118, 120

primate, 10, 17, 22, 23, 30, 43,
    44 (Table 7), 74, 131
proceptivity, 135
progestagen, 26, 136
progesterone, 11, 21, 26, 27, 30,
    33 (Table 6), 39, 136
prolactin, 8 (Table 1), 21, 23, 24,
    39
prostaglandin, 39
puberty, 6, 8 (Table 1), 14, 39, 75,
    49 (Table 9)

qualitative, 22, 43, 74, 87
    reproductive toxicity screen, 3,
        4 (Fig. 1), 6, 7, 9, 13, 18, 19
    risk assessment, 46, 100, 128,
        140
    test, 10, 71
Quantitative, 21, 25, 28, 43, 74,
    87, 121, 128
    reproductive toxicity test, 3, 4
        (Fig. 1), 7, 10, 18, 24, 55, 71
    risk, 4, 5, 32, 46, 56, 108, 110,
        140

rabbit, 43, 44 (Table 7), 46, 47
    (Table 8), 49 (Table 9), 50
    (Table 10), 51, 56, 57, 58
    (Table 11), 59, 60, 62, 70, 74,
    76, 77, 79, 81, 83, 85, 102, 105
rat, 13, 14 (Table 2), 17, 19, 20,
    22, 23, 25, 26, 32, 43, 44
    (Table 7), 47 (Table 8), 49
    (Table 9), 50 (Table 10), 51,
    56, 57, 58 (Table 11), 59-62,
    73, 74, 79, 81, 83, 85, 102,
    105, 110 (Table 12), 124, 127-
    129, 131, 133-135, 140
receptivity, 9, 124, 126, 127, 132,
    134-136
registries of birth defects, 120
radioimmunoassay, 22, 23, 31,
    81, 82, 130

reproductive capabilities, 6, 8
    (Table 1)
reproductive capacity, 62
reproductive dysfunction, 49
    (Table 9), 53, 55, 82
reproductive function, 20, 41,
    42, 53, 56-58, 137
reproductive performance, 14, 55
reproductive toxicants, 3, 6, 7, 9-
    11, 48, 52, 54, 80, 81, 86, 123,
    137
research, 2, 9-12, 49 (Table 9),
    60-62, 76, 112, 120, 121, 123,
    139, 140
reversibility, 2, 7, 26, 47 (Table 8),
    59, 81, 126, 139
risk assessment, 1, 3, 4 (Fig. 1), 7,
    11-13, 42, 52, 56, 57, 61, 69,
    86, 99, 117, 121, 123, 139
risk estimation, 2, 99, 100, 109,
    111, 112
rodent, 17, 18, 20, 27
route of administration (or
    exposure), 9, 16, 26, 27, 57, 83,
    101, 121, 130

safety factor, 9, 52, 56, 57, 110-
    112
screening system (or procedures),
    3, 4 (Fig. 1), 5-7, 14 (Table 2),
    16-18, 25, 27, 46, 47 (Table 8),
    50 (Table 10), 53, 54, 57, 61,
    62, 71, 74, 78, 79, 87, 107, 109,
    110 (Table 12), 124, 129, 131,
    137
scrotol circumference, 69, 70
semen, 41-43, 44 (Table 7), 46,
    47 (Table 8), 49, 50 (Table 10),
    51, 53-55, 58 (Table 11), 59-62,
    69, 73-79, 82, 85-87, 96
seminal
    characteristics, 60, 70, 74, 75
    collections, 46, 74, 76, 82

fluid (or plasma), 44 (Table 7),
    47 (Table 8), 49 (Table 9), 50
    (Table 10), 53, 54, 59-61, 75,
    76, 79, 80, 82
    volume, 47 (Table 8), 50 (Table 10),
    60, 74, 75, 82, 84, 96
seminiferous epithelium, 44 (Table 7),
    47 (Table 8), 48, 51, 57, 71, 74,
    75, 83, 84, 88, 93, 94, 96
Sertoli cell, 62, 71, 72, 83, 84
sexual
    behavior, 1, 8 (Table 1), 10, 20,
        25-27, 43, 62, 80, 117, 123-131,
        134-140
    dysfunction, 53, 123, 125, 137-139
    function, 26, 80, 104, 124, 137,
        138, 140
    gratification, 125, 138-140
    initative, 124-126, 131, 138
    responsiveness, 124-126, 131,
        135, 136
short-term test, 31, 62, 107-109,
    110 (Table 12)
sonography, 53
species, 7, 9, 11, 16, 17, 28, 30-32,
    43, 46, 49 (Table 9), 51, 56,
    57, 61, 69-71, 74-76, 79-81,
    100-106, 110-112, 117, 122-124,
    126, 128-131, 134, 140
sperm, 16, 41-43, 44 (Table 7),
    46, 47 (Table 8), 49 (Table 9),
    50 (Table 10), 51, 54, 59, 69,
    62, 69, 71, 72, 74-76, 78-80,
    82, 84-87, 132
    abnormalities, 60-62, 78, 85, 87
    chromatin, 62
    concentration, 41, 42, 46, 47
        (Table 8), 50 (Table 10), 72,
        76, 77, 82
    count, 42, 53, 54, 72, 76, 138
    genone, 41, 62, 85, 86
    head, 55, 62, 73, 78, 83
    maturation, 43
    morphology, 41, 42, 46, 47
        (Table 8), 50 (Table 10), 51,
        53, 55, 59-62, 73, 75, 78, 79, 84, 87

motility, 42, 43, 46, 47 (Table 8),
  50 (Table 10), 51, 53, 60, 72,
  73, 75, 77-79, 82-84, 93, 95
number, 41, 46, 47 (Table 8), 50
  (Table 10), 53, 55, 72, 76-79,
  82, 84, 85, 98
production, 42, 44 (Table 7), 51,
  54, 60, 70, 75-77, 80, 85, 94
size, 55
transport, 44 (Table 7), 47
  (Table 8), 59, 62, 70, 85
spermatid, 44 (Table 7), 47
  (Table 8), 50 (Table 10), 51,
  58, 70, 71, 83, 84
spermatocytes, 44 (Table 7), 47
  (Table 8), 49, 51, 71, 72, 83, 84
spermatogenesis, 43, 70, 71, 74,
  78, 80, 86, 94, 97
spermatogonia, 42, 44 (Table 7),
  49, 51, 59, 71
spermatozoa, 42, 46, 49 (Table 9),
  55, 60, 62, 69, 70, 72-74, 78,
  83, 85-87, 94-98
spermatozoal concentration, 42,
  76, 84
spermicidal, 79
spermiogenesis, 51
spontaneous luteinization, 32
sterility, 71, 80, 82, 86
steroid, 16, 17, 21, 28, 30, 31
  (Table 5), 32, 33 (Table 6),
  127, 136, 137
steroidogenesis, 8 (Table 1), 10,
  16, 21, 28-30, 31 (Table 5), 32,
  33 (Table 6), 39, 136, 137
structure-function, 3-7, 9, 10, 56
subchronic, 3, 48, 57
surveillance study, 52, 54, 120,
  121, 136, 137

testicular
  function, 41, 42, 46, 52-56, 58,
    60, 61, 69, 71, 72, 74, 78-80,
    82
  size, 44 (Table 7), 47 (Table 8),
    50 (Table 10), 51, 53, 54, 60,
    69, 70, 74, 84

testis, 42, 44 (Table 7), 47
  (Table 8), 49 (Table 9), 50
  (Table 10), 51, 54, 56, 69, 70,
  71, 73, 74, 79, 80, 83-85, 127,
  128, 131
testis weight, 44 (Table 7), 47
  (Table 8), 50 (Table 10), 58
  (Table 11), 70, 77, 83, 84
testosterone (T), 6, 20, 30, 33
  (Table 6), 39, 41, 47 (Table 8),
  48, 50 (Table 10), 54, 59, 61,
  62, 69, 79-84, 97, 128, 129, 131
thecol, 30, 32, 33 (Table 6)
threshold level, 2, 42, 56, 88, 103,
  110, 111, 130
thyrotropin, 23
tonometry, 49 (Table 9), 53, 60

uncertainty factor, 56
uterus (or uterine), 5, 8 (Table 1),
  13, 14 (Table 2), 18, 19, 112,
  122

vagina, 8 (Table 1), 43, 59, 74, 84,
  132, 133, 136, 138
vaginal
  opening, 5, 13, 14 (Table 2), 18,
    20
  smear, 16, 20, 58 (Table 11),
    135
validation, 7, 10, 16, 32, 46, 49
  (Table 9), 55, 84, 85, 99, 108,
  109, 112, 119, 120
vesicular gland, 47 (Table 8), 50
  (Table 10), 73, 78, 83
videotape (video), 46, 47 (Table 8),
  48, 50 (Table 10), 60, 73, 78, 82
virilization, 8 (Table 1), 40, 126

zona pellucida, 84, 86
zygote, 8 (Table 1), 104

About the Series Editor

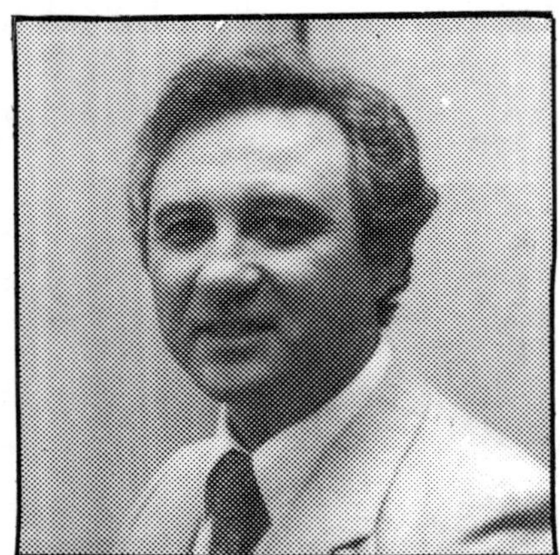

Myron A. Mehlman, Ph. D.

Dr. Myron A. Mehlman is the Director of Toxicology and Manager of the Environmental and Health Sciences Laboratory at Mobil Oil Corporation. Born in 1934, Dr. Mehlman was educated at the City College of New York (B.S. 1957), the Massachusetts Institute of Technology (Ph.D. 1964), the University of Wisconsin (Post-Doctoral Fellow, Institute for Enzyme Research, 1967), and Harvard Business School (Program for Health Systems Management, 1974). His academic appointments include Associate Professor of Biochemistry (1967-1969) at Rutgers University and Professor Biochemistry (1969-1974) at the University of Nebraska. He was appointed Adjunct Professor of Medicine at the Mt. Sinai School of Medicine in 1980.

Dr. Mehlman was Chief of Biochemical Toxicology (1972-1973) at FDA, Special Assistant for Toxicology, Environmental Affairs, and Nutrition (1973-1975) at Office of Assistant Secretary for Health, HEW, and Special Assistant for Program Planning and Evaluation, and Interagency Liaison Officer, Office of Director at National Institutes of Health (1975-1977).

In addition to serving as Chairman of the First and Second National Meetings of the American College of Toxicology, he has chaired symposia at Rutgers University, the University of Nebraska, FASEB, NIH, and the FDA. His professional memberships include the American Society of Biological Chemists, the American Physiological Society, American Institute of Nutrition, American Society for Experimental Therapeutics and Pharmacology, the American Chemical Society, the Society of Toxicology, the American College of Toxicology and the American Industrial Hygienist Society.

Dr. Mehlman is also the founding editor of the Journal of Toxicology and Environmental Health and the Journal of Environmental Pathology and Toxicology, and has been a series editor for Advances in Modern Nutrition, Advances in Modern Toxicology, Symposium on Metabolic Regulation, and Advances in Modern Environmental Toxicology. From 1977-1979 Dr. Mehlman was the first and founding president of the American College of Toxicology.

Since 1962, Dr. Mehlman has published 162 articles in the fields of biochemistry, toxicology, nutrition and human health. He has edited and co-edited approximately 18 books.